2.4.97
$19

DIMENSIONS:
VISUALLY IMPAIRED PERSONS WITH MULTIPLE DISABILITIES

Compiled and with an introduction by Jane N. Erin, Ph.D.
Department of Special Education
The University of Texas at Austin

Selected Papers from
the *Journal of Visual Impairment & Blindness*

 American Foundation for the Blind, New York

DIMENSIONS: Visually Impaired Persons with Multiple Disabilities

Selected Papers from the *Journal of Visual Impairment & Blindness*

Library of Congress Cataloging-in-Publication Data

Dimensions : visually impaired persons with multiple disabilities : selected papers from the Journal of visual impairment & blindness / compiled and with an introduction by Jane N. Erin.
    p.   cm.
  ISBN 0-89128-163-0 : $12.95
    1. Visually handicapped--Rehabilitation. 2. Blind--Rehabilitation. 3. Handicapped children--Rehabilitation.
4. Rehabilitation. I. Erin, Jane N. II. Journal of visual impairment & blindness.
HV1598.D56 1989   89-18149
362.4'18--dc20   CIP

Printed in the United States of America

Table of Contents

OPPORTUNITIES

FUTURES

Foreword

As medical and rehabilitation technologies advance, the population of blind and visually impaired individuals with multiple handicaps continues to grow. More than ever, practitioners, researchers, and educators must be well-informed about advances and research that may provide solutions to the singular problems of this population.

Collected here are articles, organized into major subject areas, that were first published in the *Journal of Visual Impairment & Blindness*. Topics range from orientation and mobility for the deaf-blind child to assessment techniques; from functional vision stimulation studies to reports on group homes. Dr. Jane Erin of the University of Texas at Austin, who compiled this collection, opens with a brief introduction, provides opening paragraphs for each section, and closes with a never before published paper addressing the future. This thorough and varied array of papers is certainly to be of use and interest to all professionals charged with working with multiply handicapped people with visual impairments.

—*William F. Gallagher*
Executive Director
American Foundation for the Blind

Introduction

Humans are orderly beings. We control life through classifying its elements: we separate the peas from the mashed potatoes, the cognitive from the perceptual, the factual from the intuitive. Placed in the appropriate conceptual container, almost any abstraction becomes manageable. The more elusive an idea, the more desperate we are to classify it.

This is demonstrated in the development of philosophies concerning the learning processes of people with multiple disabilities. These children and adults operate in the same environments as other individuals, and they experience the same life sequence. In our eagerness to explain their unique processes for gathering information, however, we are quick to categorize and label; we draw conclusions based more on the types and severity of disabilities than on variables such as motivation, experience, or temperament which regulate learning among all humans. And, when a multiply handicapped individual learns a new skill, we often give credit to some external factor instead of to the responsible individual.

In the 12 years since publication of *The Journal of Visual Impairment & Blindness* began, multiply handicapped individuals with visual impairments have been recognized as people whose capabilities and needs entitle them to full and appropriate services within the blindness system. From the provision of a continuum of educational opportunities under P.L. 94-142 to the current emphasis on supported employment options, we have witnessed a movement away from categorization and toward opportunities for individual accomplishment.

The articles included here represent a range of approaches over the last 15 years toward work with the multiply handicapped individual with a visual impairment. They are selected and arranged with attention to the fact that people, regardless of physical or mental ability, achieve the most when they discover their own potential to effect change.

—Jane N. Erin

PROCESSES

Options for continued learning throughout the lifespan have evolved to regard individual preferences, abilities, and life situations. The articles in this section exemplify changing perspectives on services to multiply handicapped visually impaired individuals.

Assessment and Programming for Blind Children with Severely Handicapped Conditions

S. E. Bourgeault; R. K. Harley; R. F. DuBose; M. B. Langley

Abstract: This paper is the second of a series of articles describing the conceptualization, implementation, and results to date of the George Peabody College for Teachers Model Center for Severely Handicapped Multi-impaired Children with Visual Impairment as a Primary Handicapping Condition.

The Diagnostic Component, one of the three major units of the Model Vision Project (MVP), is responsible for conducting comprehensive evaluations and designing prescriptive programs for children and youth served by the project. This article describes the diagnostic team's integrated approach to assessment and the procedures, resources, and prepared products the team uses in carrying out its responsibilities.

The diagnostic team consists of a core of special educators and psychologists who work together on a daily basis to carry out the assessments that will be described. When medical services are indicated, the team increases to include ancillary pediatric, orthopedic, ophthalmological personnel, and others as needed. The core members are concerned with the educational needs of the child, the family's needs in nurturing the child, and the institution's role in serving the child. The core consists of two faculty supervisors representing special education and psychology, one full-time educational diagnostician, one half-time family services worker, and one half-time psychological assistant. Practicum students from each discipline actively participate each semester.

Basic assumptions

The team operates as a well integrated unit because of its fundamental agreement on several basic issues:

1) No child is untestable: Every behavior is appropriate to some level of central nervous system functioning.

2) The most significant persons in the life of a handicapped child are his primary caregivers: Primary caregivers, usually parents, are included in every aspect of the diagnostic assessment and are supported throughout the assessment by a team member who answers questions and notes areas of concern.

3) If changes are to occur through training, primary caregivers are the most likely change agents. Team members demonstrate training and handling techniques to the parents and then supervise them and offer feedback as the parents attempt to replicate the procedures they have observed. Primary caregivers are always encouraged to develop their own methods of training that coincide with the team's recommendations of producing desired changes in the child.

4) Effective carryover of the team's recommendations into the community can best be facilitated by the local agent most responsible for the child's educational program. A member of this local agency is requested to participate in the evaluation of the child in as many sessions as possible.

5) If the written prescriptive program is to be functional for the child, it must be functional for the primary caregivers and the teacher responsible for implementing the program. The written evaluations clearly describe procedures and instruments employed during the assessment, results obtained from the procedures, the implications of the results for educational programming, and recommendations for effecting changes in the home as well as in the classroom.

6) The team's evaluation methods must continually undergo rigorous evaluation: Parents must respond to the effectiveness of the services, teachers must evaluate the effectiveness of the prescriptive program, children's behavioral changes must be evaluated through a tracking form, and the team must review its own work and its service strategies based on the feedback received.

Diagnostic sequence

The initial phase of activating the diagnostic process entailed providing information regarding the availability of the MVP's services to community agencies known to or likely to serve individuals meeting the project's admission criteria. MVP staff requested referrals from community agencies in their initial contact with them. Figure 1 illustrates the flow of diagnostic services from the referral through the reevaluation.

Referrals from local agencies and primary caregivers are received by the Project Coordinator, who records on the MVP referral form relevant data regarding the individual and his or her problems. If the referral data indicate that both visual and other handicapping conditions are present, it is directed to the Project Liaison Worker, who then screens the individual for appropriateness for MVP services. The screening process occurs in the child's home and yields developmental and visual information acquired through the use of the MVP Visual Screening Inventory. Youngsters between birth and 21 years of age manifesting severe visual impairments as well as additional severely handicapping conditions other than deafness are candidates for MVP services. The screening data of individuals not meeting service criteria are sent to the referring agency with a rationale stating why the referral was not accepted. If the youngster is not being serviced by another agency, the MVP staff recommends possible educational placements and makes the initial contacts with those agencies. After parental approval is obtained, eligible children are placed on the MVP service roster and provisionally placed in an educational unit best meeting their individual needs.

The diagnostic team established a priority evaluation system to effectively handle the large number of children awaiting diagnostic services. Individuals of preschool age receiving no services are the first to be assessed; identified individuals of school age receiving no services are next to be assessed; and identified individuals already receiving educational services are last in the priority system. The team deviates from the usual priority system to conduct emergency evaluations critical for educational placements of individuals identified as appropriate for MVP services.

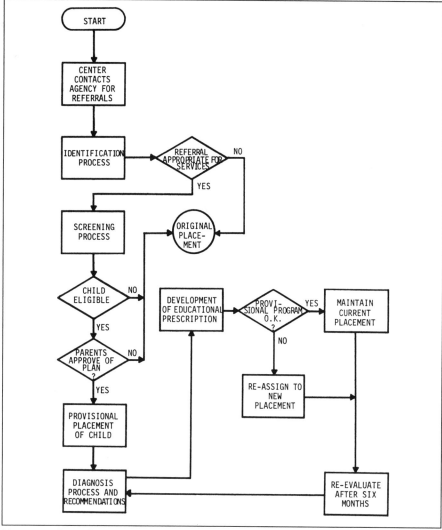

Figure 1. Flow of diagnostic services from referral to reevaluation.

Once the diagnostic assessment is completed, a written comprehensive report of the implications of the results and a prescriptive program are shared with the primary caregivers and the educational agency. If the provisional placement is verified as the best placement, then services continue at that site; if not, a reassignment is made. Between six and twelve months following the diagnostic assessment, the team reassesses the child for the purpose of changing the prescriptive program in response to his behavioral changes.

The assessment process
Three to five days are reserved for each case, depending on the complexity of the youngster's needs. The Diagnostic Coordinator prepares a schedule delineating team members responsible for the case and specific times when various components of the evaluation will occur, and distributes it to all team members, child

care participants, the child's primary caregivers, and his local educational agency. The assessment takes place in the youngster's home, classroom, individual testing rooms in the Child Study Center, and in medical offices, as well as any environmental setting relevant to the prescriptive program. The major goal of the diagnostic team is to prepare a functional assessment that for each child yields an individualized prescriptive program that can be integrated into his curriculum.

Parent interview
In keeping with the team's belief in the importance of the family unit, an interview is conducted with the child's major caregivers, most frequently his parents. The interview yields information essential to the diagnostic process, including a family history, a review of current family milieu, an overview of how the child fits into his home environment, the impres-

sions of the child as seen by the parents and siblings, and statements by the parents of their needs in relation to the child and their goals for the child. Contact between the parent liaison worker and the family is daily during the assessment process; however, more formal interviews are limited to one or two sessions.

Psychological assessment
The usefulness of measurements of mental abilities through psychological testing of individuals functioning on an infantile level has been questioned (Cronback, 1960; Geoffeney, Henderson, & Butler, 1971; Vander Veer & Schweid, 1974). If the administration of such tests produced nothing more than IQ scores, this team would not use them. However, this team's documented experience with severely handicapped children indicates that mental measures of this population are highly reliable predictors of mental development (DuBose, 1977). Mental measures obtained by this team provide highly functional information about the child's cognitive processes, add support for information acquired by other team members, and yield psychosocial data for the evaluation.

Administration of an entire psychological test according to standardized procedures is seldom possible when assessing severely handicapped children whose vision is only one of their handicapping conditions. Team psychologists frequently administer selected subtests and items from the scales they have found to be most effective in obtaining information about the child's cognitive functioning. Instruments most frequently used in the psychological assessment by the MVP psychologists are the Bayley Scales of Mental Development (Bayley, 1969), the Infant Intelligence Scale (Cattell, 1940), the Merrill Palmer Scale of Mental Abilities (Stutsman, 1948), the McCarthy Scales of Children's Abilities (McCarthy, 1972), the Stanford-Binet, and the WISC-R. The psychologists have carefully adapted items when possible, such as substituting materials with sound elements for visual items. Although they are aware of the departure from standardized norms, the psychologists have provided valuable information from these adaptions that would not have been obtained if the items had been omitted.

The educational assessment
The educational assessment provides data essential to the prescriptive program. Emphasis is placed on determining the child's developmental level of functioning in adaptive, language, motor, social, self-care,

and visual behaviors. Equally important are notations of his learning style and the material and situational characteristics that best elicit the child's potential and enhance his ability to function successfully in his environment. Kiernan and DuBose (1974) have documented the importance of the medium in the assessment of multiply handicapped children.

Motor behavior
The majority of the children served by the MVP have neurological dysfunction, necessitating the use of instruments for assessing reflexes, basic postural reactions, and early motoric milestones. Scales most frequently used have been Fiorentino's Reflex Testing Chart (1963), the Bayley Scales of Motor Development (1969), and guidelines on the development of motor skills in blind children provided by Adelson and Fraiberg (1974). More in-depth assessments of fine and gross motor skills are provided by the Peabody Developmental Motor Scales (Folio & DuBose, 1974), the Frostig Movement Skills Battery (Opert, 1972), while the Peabody Mobility Scales (Harley, Wood, & Merbler, 1975) and the Body-Image of Blind Children (Cratty & Sams, 1968) are used to obtain supplemental information regarding the child's mobility and body image concepts.

Language behaviors
Two different methods are required for assessing language in severely handicapped children, as the majority of the MVP population is nonverbal. Adequate understanding of the meaning of their communication efforts must entail assessment of the prerequisite behaviors essential for the development of symbolic language. Indeed, the implications of the way nonverbal children interact with people and objects through facial and body gestures are significant in arriving at a developmental level. Tools used in the assessment of nonverbal communication skills in multiply handicapped children are a measure developed by this project, and the Inner Language Scale (Branston & DuBose, 1974). Most valuable for understanding nonverbal communication behaviors have been sources from the literature (Morehead & Morehead, 1975; Phillips, 1969; Robbins, 1971).

The second form of language assessment encompasses information regarding phonological, morphological, semantic, and syntactical structures. The limitations imposed on instruments by the severe visual impairments of the children have narrowed the selection of functional scales. Most frequently used instruments include the Receptive-Expressive-Emergent Language Scale (Bzoch & League, 1970), the Receptive-Expressive Language Assessment for the Visually Impaired (Raynor, 1975), the Environmental Pre-language Battery (Horstmeier & MacDonald, 1975), the Environmental Language Inventory (MacDonald & Nickols, 1974), and Developmental Sentence Scoring and Sentence Types outlined by Lee (1974).

Cognitive-adaptive skills
A variety of procedures are used in the cognitive-adaptive assessment to determine strengths and weakness in the child's abilities. Adapted for use with blind children, the Developmental Activities Screening Inventory (DASI) (DuBose & Langley, 1977) is used to obtain general information regarding the child's cognitive, communicative, and fine motor abilities. The DASI provides valuable insights into the types of techniques and procedures that will be most effective in eliciting the child's maximum potential. The cognitive-adaptive assessment attempts to discover where the child is developmentally in areas of sensory-motor schemas, discrimination, association, short- and long-term memory, spatial serial relationships, deductive, inductive, and quantitative reasoning, and generalization abilities. Tools used for the assessment of children functioning on a preschool level have stemmed from Piagetian formats such as the Uzgiris-Hunt Scales (Uzgiris & Hunt, 1975) and the Infant Cognitive Development Scale (Mehrabian & Williams, 1971). The Learning Accomplishment Profile (Sanford, 1975) and Haeussermann's psychoeducational procedures (1958) have been adapted for use with children functioning on levels from two to six years. Instruments that have yielded valuable cognitive information on higher functioning verbal children have been the McCarthy Scales of Children's Abilities (1972), the Basic Concept Inventory (Englemann, 1967), the Pupil Record of Educational Behavior (Cheves, 1971), and the Detroit Tests of Learning Aptitude (Baker & Leland, 1967). Subtests from all these scales may be administered nonverbally.

Social/self-care skills
Achievement of some independence in caring for basic self-care needs is a major goal in educational programs for severely handicapped children. Emphasis is placed on detailed evaluation of the youngster's eating, dressing, toileting, and grooming behaviors, although social interactions with adults, peers, and toys also play a role in the socialization assessment. Scales that have provided the most detailed information on self-care skills include the Maxfield-Buchholz Scales of Social Maturity for Preschool Blind Children (1957), the Lakeland Village Adaptive Behavior Grid (1976), the Cain-Levine Social Competency Scale (Cain, Levine, & Elzey, 1963), the TRM Profile (DiNola, Kaminsky, & Sternfield, 1973), and guidelines from the Wabash Guide to Early Developmental Training (Tilton, Liska, & Bourland, 1972).

Social-emotional scales valuable in acquiring information about the youngster's social interactions, initiative, and independence in social situations as well as his self-control are the Bayley Infant Behavior Record (Bayley, 1969), the Adaptive Behavior Scales (Nihira, Foster, Shelhaas, & Leland, 1974), and the social adjustment subtests from the Detroit Tests of Learning Aptitude (Baker & Leland, 1967).

Knowledge of the youngster's general functioning level and his ability to comprehend language, attend to a task, manipulate materials, and cooperate and maintain self-control in social situations provides the evaluator with a sound basis for determining prevocational skills and readiness to participate in work-skill activities.

Summary
During the final days of the diagnostic process, the Diagnostic Coordinator convenes the personnel involved in the assessment and discusses the prescriptive needs of the youngster. Each team member is responsible for writing the report and the prescription for his or her respective area. The prescriptive emerges from the diagnostic findings, and trial implementation is a part of the educational assessment.

The product is a detailed plan for individual instructional services. This final product is summarized orally at the final staff meeting and written in detail in the comprehensive assessment report. Copies are made available to persons designated by the primary caregivers as the recipients. Follow-up is carried out through tracking from reports and direct service contacts. Children can be reassessed after six months. The reassessment is a condensed evaluation for the purpose of confirming the placement and making prescriptive changes in the curriculum.

Dissemination of products, procedures, and training

A major commitment of all the BEH-funded model centers is to produce a model for services that can be replicated throughout a state. The diagnostic unit has developed and distributed the Visual Screening Inventory as a screening tool to be used by local educational agents in identifying youngsters in need of services because of major visual anomalies. Also available from the unit is a list of assessment tools found most useful with severely handicapped blind children. Procedures and products have been shared through workshops and inservice training in residential, public, and private schools throughout the country.

The diagnostic staff has initiated a local training model for meeting the needs of local youngsters after the MVP completes its work as a federally funded unit. The diagnostic agent most likely to serve each youngster at a future time is requested to observe the youngster's assessment and begin to take over responsibilities related to his assessment needs. Agents are later invited to participate in a workshop program to acquire more intensive practical knowledge of the model advocated by this team.

This article has described the model and procedures used by the diagnostic team of the Model Visual Project. The model includes the families and local educational agents as major components of the assessment process. The procedures include formal and informal investigations that culminate in a functional individualized educational program for each individual.

References

Adelson, E. & Fraiberg, S. (1974). Gross motor development in infants blind from birth. *Child Development,* **45,** 114-126.

Baker, H.J. & Leland, B. (1967). *Detroit Tests of Learning Aptitude.* Indianapolis: Bobbs-Merrill.

Bayley, N. (1969). *The Bayley Scales of Infant Development.* New York: Psychological Corporation.

Branston, M.B. & DuBose, R.F. (1974). *Inner Language Scale.* Nashville, TN: George Peabody College for Teachers.

Bzoch, K. & League, R. (1970). *The Receptive-Expressive-Emergent Language Scale.* Gainesville, FL: The Anbinga Press.

Cain, L.F., Levine, S., & Elzey, F. (1963). *Cain-Levine Social Competency Scale.* Palo Alto, CA: Consulting Psychologists Press.

Cattell, P. (1940). *The Infant Intelligence Scale.* New York: Psychological Corporation.

Cheves, R. (1971). *P.R.E.B. Pupil Record of Educational Behavior.* Boston: Teaching Resources.

Cratty, B.J. & Sams, F.A. (1968). *The body-image of blind children.* New York: American Foundation for the Blind.

Cronback, L. (1960). *Essentials of psychological testing.* New York: Harper & Row.

DiNola, A.J., Kaminsky, B.P., & Sternfield, A.E. (1973). *T.M.R. Performance Profile for the Severely and Moderately Retarded.* Ridgefield, NJ: Educational Performance Associates.

DuBose, R.J. (in press). The predictive value of infant scales with deaf-blind children. *American Journal of Mental Deficiency.*

DuBose, R.J., & Langley, M.B. (1977). *The Development Activities Screening Inventory.* Boston: Teaching Resources.

Englemann, S. (1967). *The Basic Concept Inventory.* Chicago: Follett Educational Corporation, 1967.

Fiorentino, M.R. (1963). *Reflex testing methods of evaluating C.N.S. development.* Springfield, IL: Charles C Thomas.

Folio, R.F. & DuBose, R.F. (1974). *Peabody Developmental Motor Scales.* IMRD Behavioral Research Institute, Monograph No. 25, George Peabody College, Nashville, TN.

Geoffeney, B., Henderson, N.B., & Butler, B.V. (1971). Negro-white, male-female: Eight month developmental scores compared with developmental problems. *Child Development,* **42,** 596-604.

Haeussermann, E. (1958). *Developmental potential for preschool children.* New York: Grune & Stratton.

Harley, R.K., Wood, T.A., & Merbler, J.B. (1975). *Peabody Orientation and Mobility Scales,* George Peabody College for Teachers, Nashville, TN, Revised experimental edition (final publication draft) in preparation.

Horstmeier, D.S. & MacDonald, J.D. (1975). *Environmental Pre-Language Battery.* Columbus, OH: Nisonger Center, Ohio State University.

Kiernan, D.W. & DuBose, R.F. (1974). Assessing the cognitive development of preschool deaf-blind. *Education of the Visually Handicapped,* **6,** 103-105.

Lakeland Village Adaptive Behavior Grid (Experimental Version) (1976). Washington: Lakeland Village.

Lee, L.L. (1974). *Developmental sequence analysis: A grammatical assessment procedure for speech and language clinicians.* Evanston, IL: Northwestern University Press.

McCarthy, D. (1972). *McCarthy Scales of Children's Abilities.* New York: The Psychological Corporation.

MacDonald, J.D. & Nickols, M. (1974). *Environmental Language Inventory.* Colum-bus, OH: Nisonger Clinic, Ohio State University.

Maxfield, K.E. & Buchholz, S.B. (1957). *A Social Maturity Scale for Blind Preschool Children.* New York: American Foundation for the Blind.

Mehrabian, A. & Williams, M. (1971). Piagetian measures of cognitive development up to age two. *Journal of Psycholinguistic Research,* **1,** 113-116.

Morehead, D.M. & Morehead, A.E. (1976). *Normal and deficient child language.* Baltimore: University Park Press.

Nihira, K., Foster, R., Shelhaas, M., & Leland, H. (1974). *Adaptive Behavior Scale Manual.* Washington, DC: American Association on Mental Deficiency.

Orpet, R.E. (1972). *The Frostig Movement Skills Battery.* Palo Alto, CA: Consulting Psychologists Press.

Phillips, J.L. (1969). *The origins of intellect: Piaget's theory.* San Francisco: W.H. Freeman.

Raynor, S. (1975). *Receptive Expressive Language Assessment for the Visually Impaired 0-6.* Mason, MI: Outreach Project.

Robbins, N. (1971). *The teaching of a manual sign as a diagnostic tool with deaf-blind children.* In Fourth International Conference on Deaf-Blind Children. Watertown, MA: Perkins School for the Blind.

Sanford, A.R. (1975). *Learning Accomplishment Profile.* Winston-Salem, NC: Kaplan School Supply Corp.

Spivack, G. & Spotts, J. (1966). *Devereux Behavior Rating Scales.* Devon, PA: The Devereux Foundation.

Stutsman, R. (1948). *Merrill-Palmer Scale of Mental Tests.* Chicago: C.H. Stoelting.

Tilton, J.R., Liska, D.C., & Bourland, J.D. (eds.) (1972). *Guide to early developmental training.* Lafayette, IN: Wabash Center Sheltered Workshop.

Uzgiris, I.C. & Hunt, J. McV. (1975). *Assessment in infancy: Ordinal scales of psychological development.* Urbana, IL: University of Illinois.

Vander Veer, B. & Schweid, E. (1974). Infant assessment: Stability of mental functioning in young retarded children. *American Journal of Mental Deficiency,* **79.**

S.E. Bourgeault, associate professor of special education, co-director of the Model Vision Project, and director of field services; R.K. Harley, professor of special education, co-director of the Model Vision Project; R.F. DuBose, associate professor of special education, coordinator of the diagnostic and evaluation component; M.B. Langley, educational diagnostician, George Peabody College for Teachers, Nashville, Tennessee.

Combining Specialties to Serve Low Functioning, Visually/Physically Impaired Children

D. Cech; A. Pitello

Abstract: This article explores the impact of combining a vision specialist's abilities with those of a physical therapist when working with low functioning, preschool, visually and physically impaired children. Individually prescribed programs are cited to demonstrate the utility of a multidisciplinary approach. The authors view this article as an exploratory starting point for educators for further program development serving low incidence students.

A multidisciplinary approach was used to serve visually and physically impaired children in a preschool program. Aware of an incoming preschool population of these children, public school educators worked with the regional special education cooperative to design a program that would provide a low student-teacher ratio with emphasis on visual programming. It was hoped that, by providing the services of both a vision specialist and a physical therapist, a program to help to meet the extraordinary needs of these children could be developed.

The children attended the program six hours a day, five days a week. Diagnostic visual assessment, preschool experiences, and self-help activities were an integral part of the school day. In addition, they received individualized physical therapy for approximately 45 minutes, three times a week. Emphasis was placed on giving the classroom teacher a clear understanding of the objectives of each child's therapy, including handling techniques, positioning, and suggestions for feeding, so that the best, consistent, environmental management could be provided throughout the school day.

Two of the children in the program serve as examples of how the multidisciplinary approach was developed. One, a boy aged 3½, had had anophthalmia from birth with severe developmental motor delays. The other, a girl aged 2½, was exotropic with visual acuity unknown and, in addition, had quadriplegic cerebral palsy. Neither child could walk or talk and both had feeding problems. Both were functioning below a six-month level of development.

Encouraging environmental exploration

The boy did not respond to his environment. Tactile exploration was limited to putting things in his mouth, particularly his own fingers. He uttered only occasional self-stimulating sounds. Left unattended, he favored lying on the floor. Sitting was an insecure position and not maintained for any length of time, and crawling, kneeling, standing, and walking were beyond him.

As he did not have the muscle tone, head control, trunk control, or balance skills necessary for motor activity, he found it easier to move in abnormal patterns. In addition, his blindness prevented him from imitating the movements of other people. His program was designed to build basic skills that would be necessary for later sensory development and to help to compensate for his visual and physical impairments.

As progress took place in these areas, demands upon him were expanded to include movement through space and broader exploration of the environment. Consistent repetitive physical guidance was given in all motor activities to insure a normal progression of motor development.

As a result of the intensive nine-month intervention program, the child became more highly motivated and initiated more environmental exploration. He was now actively grasping, patting, banging, and manipulating objects. Verbalization became more "situation-appropriate" and had more inflection. He was now able to assume and maintain a sitting position, move to and from kneeling, stand at furniture, and walk with hands held. With much encouragement and assistance, he was beginning to crawl for short distances.

The girl presented a completely different management problem. Cerebral palsy affected muscle control throughout her body, including oral and visual mechanisms. She was nonverbal and functioning as a blind child.

Several things were noticed about the child's visual functioning. When unattended, she would cover one eye and visually explore her surroundings with the uncovered eye. There appeared to be no central fixation, and there were no tracking abilities present, which was not surprising with her level of motor dysfunction.

Two factors, hypertonicity and some pathological reflex activity (excessive tone, tension, or activity), made it impossible for the child to control her head, her trunk, or her movements. She was unable to lift her hands together at the midline, or sit without shoulder and trunk support.

When verbalization was attempted, hypertonicity caused jaw thrusting which limited oral expression to squeals, shrieks, and vowel sounds. Eating skills such as chewing, swallowing, and lip closure were difficult and poorly coordinated.

The only movements she made were dominated by hypertonicity and were, therefore, abnormal and would significantly limit progress in motor development and cause deformities. It was also felt that arrested motor development could be inhibiting her intellectual ability and therefore might lead to functional retardation.

Improving muscle tone

Abnormal muscle tone appeared to be the key factor in all areas of development. Careful analysis was made of her muscle tone while she was in different positions. The effects of hypertonicity on performance in different activities were also scrutinized.

Based on these observations, a program centered around positioning and handling techniques was designed to inhibit abnormal muscle tone. The normalization of muscle tone allowed the child to experience a more normal sensation of movement, with potential for better motor and intellectual development.

Consistency was an important part of her program. For the positioning and handling techniques to be most effective, they had to be a fundamental part of her daily routine. All school personnel involved with the child, as well as her family, worked to maintain this consistency. This was no small task, since carrying, dressing, picking her up, structuring learning, playing, developing language, and eating were all a part of the routine.

For example, when lying on her back, hypertonicity caused her head to be tilted backwards, limiting the visual field. Her arms were fixed at her sides and bent at the elbows, with her hands clenched at her shoulders. She lacked the ability to raise her arms off the floor, making it impossible to reach for toys, play with her hands, or explore her surroundings.

A rolled towel was placed under her head in an attempt to break up the hypertonicity. It was also necessary to flex her hips and knees routinely to control the excessive muscle tone. These adaptations allowed her to experience a more normal sensation of movement and better interaction with her surroundings. She began to move her arms more freely, reaching for objects and bringing her hands together at the midline. The opportunity was now provided for her to explore visually what went on in front of her rather than behind her. Because her head was brought forward, she was no longer locked into an upward or backward field of vision.

Nine months of consistent programming resulted in the girl's learning to control her head well enough to turn toward a noise source. She could focus momentarily and showed some ability to track an object by moving her whole head. She could now raise her head and turn it from side to side while in a prone position, and was also beginning to reach for and grasp objects. Support was only needed at the midback and hips for sitting, as head, shoulder, and upper trunk control had improved.

Improvement in head control led to more normal oral-motor functioning in both speech and feeding. The variety of verbalizations had increased to include "ba," "ma," "te," "p," "de," and "da" sounds. The intensity and inflection of her sounds had expanded. She was now able to take food from a spoon, bite, chew, and swallow with considerable success. Drinking continued to be somewhat of a problem.

People who knew the child before her placement in the program recognized the significance of the gains achieved in the nine-month period.

The complexities of the children's handicaps were such that neither child could be viewed primarily as a physically impaired child or a visually impaired child.

Setting apart the boy's blindness, his program would have included efficient movement through space; self-help skills; increased environmental awareness through auditory, kinesthetic, olfactory, and tactile modalities; and socialization. But learning potential was complicated by blindness and motor delays, and work on his program could not begin. Lack of sufficient muscle tone, poor head and trunk control, and inadequate balance skills placed him at a developmental level below that necessary to achieve the aforementioned program goals. Emphasis in his program had to be on development of beginning motor skills.

Effectiveness of dual-discipline approach
By combining the motor development background of the physical therapist and the knowledge of the developmental limitations of blindness offered by the vision specialist, a multidisciplinary program was implemented. While separate vision and motor programs are seemingly effective, the dual-discipline approach allowed the child to achieve goals without nonessential or counter-productive steps. It is my feeling that coexistent rather than coordinated programming is prone to such nonessential or counter-productive steps.

It was apparent that a similar course of action was vital in working with the girl. Remediation for her visual dysfunction could not be dealt with successfully until her head control was improved. When she could control her head in space, she would have sufficient stability for visual development. The physical therapist worked with her to develop head control. As progress was made, the therapist and teacher utilized their skills to develop positioning techniques designed to provide maximum opportunity for visual development.

We approached the children's problems each from a different perspective. By sharing these perspectives, learning was fostered and we gained insight into one another's professional viewpoints and experiences. The integrated approach led to a "total-child" program design, providing the children with a more complete foundation on which to build future learning experiences.

To serve multiply handicapped children, professionals from many fields must learn to work cooperatively, sharing their expertise and experiences openly. Only by such cooperation and sharing will multiply handicapped children receive a comprehensive individualized program, uniquely suited to their educational and physical needs.

Donna Cech, R.P.T., physical therapist, Northwestern Illinois Association, DeKalb, IL; Ardis Pitello, M.A., preschool teacher of visually impaired children.

The Blind and Visually Handicapped Mentally Retarded: Suggestions for Intervention in Infancy

A.A. Mori; J.E. Olive

Abstract: This article presents a rationale for implementing early transdisciplinary intervention in behalf of blind and visually handicapped, mentally retarded infants. The program stresses normal developmental goals, a holistic approach to the child and family, and techniques for enhancing the development of the child's reflexes and gross motor skills; sensory, cognitive, and fine motor skills; language; and affective personality and independence. The roles of professionals and parents receive special emphasis.

Experimentation and research in the field of special education over the past two decades have provided educators with growing evidence that a number of techniques and approaches are productive as early intervention strategies on behalf of handicapped infants. These techniques are usually based on developmental models and can be applied in areas of physical, occupational, and speech therapy, as well as sensory and cognitive stimulation. Moreover, progress has been made in developing supportive services that will aid parents in helping their child develop appropriate affective behaviors early in life.

Because of the efforts of practitioners in a variety of fields, four basic principles have emerged that apply to the needs of the whole child, whatever his handicap. It is also possible to foresee certain problems that may arise in caring for multiply handicapped infants. This article describes how these principles can be applied in an effective and efficient early intervention program designed to help blind and mentally retarded infants reach their highest potential as whole persons. These same principles can be applied in intervention programs dealing with other handicapping conditions.

In the case of special education in early childhood, effective intervention begins with the earliest possible diagnosis of the infant's condition. Concurrently, supportive services and programs of intervention must be initiated for the parents without delay.

Crisis of discovery

Our research suggests that the first principle of effective intervention on behalf of handicapped infants and their parents is immediate response. During the crisis that is precipitated when the parents learn of an infant's handicap, intervention must be initiated in a matter of days, not weeks or months. Efficient, empathic services begin with a valid diagnosis; an appropriate, transdisciplinary program of intervention; and appropriate supportive services for the family.

Diagnosis and transdisciplinary programming

The infant's condition must be analyzed immediately and as thoroughly as possible. This analysis should include a neurological examination as well as a thorough physical evaluation (Cratty, 1971), and the infant's overall reactions and affective characteristics must also be carefully evaluated and documented (Brazelton, 1975). The diagnosis must then be shared with a transdisciplinary team of practitioners (Chase, 1975) consisting of individuals who have been trained in the developmental principles of early cognitive learning processes, the therapeutic techniques required by the child's condition, and counseling skills and experience related to the family's needs. The program of intervention that these practitioners design should be initiated as soon as the infant's health permits. Initially, the educator, therapist, and counselor should work together to ensure that the parents receive crisis counseling and that the infant's pro-

gram is securely established. Thereafter, the educator can carry out the program and consult the original transdisciplinary team regularly for reevaluation as well as additional training, if necessary.

Intervention during the crisis period should be home-based. In other words, the educator (and therapists, if required) should go to the home or hospital every day until the parents or nursing staff are able to deliver appropriate services to the child. If the infant is hospitalized for an extended period, the educator can train the parents by using a doll. He can also discuss problems that the parents will encounter, allay the parents' fears, and strengthen their self-confidence. This strategy not only helps parents adjust more positively to the situation but also encourages happier affective relationships between parents and infants.

Volunteers such as friends of the family, relatives, and parents of children with similar handicaps can also be trained to help parents work effectively with their infant (Richards, 1971). This is especially valuable when the infant's condition requires hours of daily therapeutic work.

Counseling and supportive services

According to DuBose (1976), the single most influential factor in a blind child's development is the parents' ability to accept and cope with the dilemma the child presents. Typically, parents of a defective baby question their masculinity or femininity; some find the infant frightening and repulsive (Fraiberg, 1975). These reactions, combined with confusion and a socially conditioned sense of guilt, may cause parents to avoid interacting with the baby for prolonged periods. Thus, intervention must be initiated immediately (Bornstein, 1974; Froyd, 1973; Connelly, 1969; Warnick, 1969). Fraiberg, Smith, and Adelson (1969) and Burlingham (1969) stress the need to involve and help the father. Intensive crisis counseling (Parad, 1975) for six weeks during the initial crisis seems to be the most effective and relevant method of helping families that are suffering the despair of "losing" the expected infant and are facing all the uncertainties involved in rearing a handicapped child. After this intensive period, additional counseling can be given when required.

During the initial six weeks, parents can also be introduced to the educational program designed for their infant and should be encouraged to participate with professionals in the child's program as soon as possible. As their confidence increases, their opinions and desires must be integrated into the program.

Parents of blind children will find the following reading materials helpful at this time: *Get a wiggle on* and *Move it* (Raynor & Drouillard, 1975, 1977), *Our blind children: Growing and learning with them* (Lowenfeld, 1964), and selected articles in the *Journal of Visual Impairment & Blindness*. Lowenfeld's book is still a standard source for learning about the challenges of raising a blind child.

Parents should be advised that a blind infant often encounters difficult periods of growth and development (Fraiberg, Smith & Adelson, 1969). For example, he will walk later than the normal child. If he suffers the additional handicaps of mental retardation and cerebral palsy, he will develop even more slowly and require concentrated intervention. Any program that challenges these multiple problems may seem especially encouraging to parents during the first year.

Lairy and Harrison-Covello (1973) advise professionals to encourage parents to avoid being overly protective. The baby needs to be taken out into the world and be exposed to life, language, touch, taste, and sound. Despite his handicaps, he needs to be bounced and cuddled, tossed and hugged by parents, other relatives, and friends. An infant who lacks this stimulation often withdraws and then objects strenuously to changes in lifestyle. Of course, the advice of physicians and therapists must be considered if additional conditions impair the baby's health.

Because the cost of caring for a handicapped infant can be a heavy burden, the parents may need financial aid. Thus, counselors should be familiar with local, state, and national organizations that provide funds for this purpose. They should also be familiar with the bureaucratic red tape that is frustrating to anyone but is especially so to individuals who are experiencing severe stress. In addition, parents who have already gone through and learned to cope with this tragedy may be far more helpful to parents who are still in shock than are professionals, because they are an example of successful adjustment, hope, and useful experience.

Parents need to build rewarding lives for themselves in addition to the hours of work and discouraging times they face with the baby. Counselors need to remind parents to take one day at a time; they will adjust, there will be good times and their infant will, in one way or another, reward

their efforts. Counselors can also help parents find suitable respite care so that the family can develop a lifestyle that suits the needs of all members.

Professionals must use sensitivity when dealing with parents. All responsible family members are entitled to reports concerning diagnosis and programming (Gorham, 1975). Many parents will need to be involved in their child's program, even to the point of working for legislation and public education that will result in greater normalizing possibilities for their child and a more accepting society when their child nears adulthood.

Since the blind or partially sighted young child may benefit greatly from a professional preschool program, parents may wish to place him in a good preschool program for normal youngsters. If this is impossible, parents can band together and develop their own program. The following sources may be helpful in this area: *Move it* (Raynor & Drouillard, 1977), *Mainstreaming preschoolers: Children with visual handicaps* (Contract Research Corporation, 1977), "How to play with your partially sighted child" (Barry, 1973), *Preschool learning activities for the visually impaired child; A guide for parents* (Instructional Materials Center), *Our blind children* (Lowenfeld, 1964), *Blind preschool* (Taylor, 1974), *Project FAITH curriculum for infant learning* (Mori & Olive, 1976; see "Sensory-cognitive goals phase V"), *Project FAITH parent handbook* (Olive, 1976; "Unit activities, discovery, manipulation and patterns").

Developmental program for blind and multiply handicapped infants

A program designed to meet the needs of infants with a variety of handicapping conditions should be based on the principles of normal human development. When dealing with children whose capacity to learn is impaired, however, it is important to stress the skills to be developed rather than the normal age at which infants reach developmental milestones.

Another principle of successful programming is that the developmental guidelines allow for the development of the *total* child as an individual. Thus, the program must include a variety of teaching procedures that focus on the development of: 1) reflexes and gross motor development, 2) sensory, cognitive, and fine motor skills, 3) language, 4) personality and social skills, and 5) independence. Ongoing assessment and evaluation must be an integral part of such programming.

Recent efforts to design this type of flexible program include *Project FAITH curriculum for infant learning* (Mori & Olive, 1976) and *Project FAITH parent handbook* (Olive, 1976). The curricula described in these sources take into account the blind infant's altered developmental course, which, according to Fraiberg, Smith, and Adelson (1969), requires certain alterations in developmental goals.

General suggestions
The following general suggestions are useful when designing developmental programs for blind infants:

• "Bonding" between infant and parents should be established as quickly as possible (Fraiberg, Smith, & Adelson, 1969).

• The child's primitive reflexes should be stimulated to increase his memory of the processes involved (Brown, 1977). This process, however, should be supervised by a physician and a physical therapist because some primitive reflexes interfere with more advanced developmental skills (Evans & Summer, 1975).

• Two major goals are to help the child develop a positive self-image and the sense of independence that will make that positive self-concept a reality (Fraiberg, Smith, & Adelson, 1969; McClennen, 1969; Carolan, 1973). In other words, a blind child needs to be protected from those who would overprotect him and "make him a blind man" (DuBose, 1976).

• Stimulation of all senses—touch, taste, smell, and hearing—should be integrated into each child's program. This lays the foundation for later cognitive development as well as a sound sense of self-awareness. Visual stimulation for white or colored light can also be included in the sensory program when appropriate (caution is necessary if the infant's condition includes seizures).

• Many "blindisms" are currently viewed as a blind child's way of stimulating himself when bored. Some are viewed as mere mannerisms that are the result of the child's inability to visualize normal cultural postures. Cratty (1971) and Taylor (1974) suggest that providing more activities for the child will alleviate the former, while ongoing early conditioning of better postures will curtail the latter.

• Language development appears to have two aspects. First, family members should learn to recognize the minute gestures that the blind infant uses to communicate with others (Fraiberg, 1975). For example, if an infant becomes quiet when someone enters the room, the parent may misinterpret what is actually an attending device as the baby's rejection of them (Froyd, 1973). Second, adults should talk to the infant often and in a meaningful way and reinforce his responses (Froyd, 1973).

The following suggestions are useful when designing a program for the blind infant who is mentally retarded:

- Parents and educators will usually spend more time in teaching skills if the skill is broken down into its simplest parts.
- Because it is often difficult to find appropriate rewards for infants who seem unresponsive, parents and educators should be imaginative and learn to recognize the baby's subtle indications of satisfaction or pleasure (Parker, 1971; Stockmeyer, 1972). Sometimes a back rub, cooing sounds, a hug, or a bell is useful as a reinforcer or reward.
- Simple, direct, and frequently repeated language is useful when working with mentally retarded infants. Too much or meaningless language may interfere with conceptualization (Moss & Mayer, 1975).
- Physical therapists should be involved directly in all work on infant reflexes and gross motor skills because of possible cerebral involvement. Certain techniques are more applicable to specific conditions, such as cerebral palsy and the attending problems of muscle tone.
- Stimulation of the senses is important. But if it aggravates the child's seizures or cerebral palsy, it should be modified in intensity and duration and be followed by relaxation techniques tailored to the child's specific needs. Because tactile information seems to be more easily forgotten than visual information (Moss & Mayer, 1975), deliberate stimulation of the infant's other senses should be carried out as often as is feasible.
- Sensory stimuli such as brushing, bell-ringing, patting, and making verbal noises should be in a rhythmical, non-monotonous pattern such as a long, short; short, long. This technique tends not only to enhance development of memory, and cognitive discrimination (Carolan, 1973), as well as attention span but also helps lay a foundation for the spatial, temporal, and numerical concepts that are the mentally retarded adult's primary deficits (Moss & Mayer, 1975).

Reflexes and gross motor skills
Voss (1972) states that "a method of treatment will be successful only if it is grounded in development of normal motor behavior, if it has a firm basis in neurophysiology, and if it includes procedures that will hasten motor learning by providing appropriate stimuli and appropriate degrees of stress." Given these criteria for success, a reliable and effective program for developing infant reflexes and gross motor skills must be understood by all those who work with the child. The following suggestions must be carefully prescribed by physicians and professional therapists and should be introduced at the appropriate time for the individual child.

Memory trace is established best through visual and motor activity (Brown, 1977). Therefore, when visual input is weak or absent, the patterns of primitive motor reflexes should be exploited.

Range-of-motion exercises, massage (Leboyer, 1976), and techniques for improving tone (Bobath, 1972) and strengthening muscles can be combined with sensory stimulation and the rhythmic patterning described in the previous section. Again, caution must be exercised if the infant's condition includes cerebral palsy, seizures, or pinched nerves.

Because hydrotherapy is relaxing for some infants (LeBoyer, 1976), it may be well to introduce reflex stimulation and exercise programs while the infant is calm and enjoying a period of play in tepid water. Before implementing this technique, however, the therapist or parent should consult a physician in regard to the infant's general health and whether the navel is healed sufficiently. Young children who can swim may enjoy playing in the water; "Swimmies" and inner tubes add to the fun.

Blind infants seem to dislike being placed in the prone position (Fraiberg, Smith, & Adelson, 1969). But because this position is important for strengthening the neck muscles, it should be made more entertaining. This can often be accomplished by dangling sound toys or bells near the infant's head or hands, which will encourage him to turn his head. Fraiberg, Smith, and Adelson (1969) suggest placing the baby in the prone position across an adult's lap, head and arms on the adult's leg, and the feet resting on the couch.

As Fraiberg (1975) points out, a blind infant may not begin creeping until he has developed the ability to reach out for an object that emits a sound.

Once the child does begin to crawl, however, the home obviously must be "child-proofed." Parents must exercise special care to see that he is not discouraged by too many bumps and falls. Guards must be put across stairs, pointed sharp edges on furniture should be covered with foam rubber. Cratty (1971) believes adults should occasionally crawl around with the child so that they will become familiar with the environment in which the child must develop mobility, self-confidence, and trust. In other words, they should arrange the environment so that the child becomes a "winner." When the child walks with confidence and indicates an ability to cooperate with others, siblings can be trained to guide him (Napier, 1974; Wardell, 1976).

Sensory, cognitive, and fine motor skills
A program for developing sensory, cognitive, and fine motor skills must help the infant attain two goals: a valid body-image and sense of self and the mechanisms required for learning. Umsted (1975) insists that in the case of blind infants, "tactile and auditory adaptations to environments are necessary as early as possible in life."

As suggested earlier, brushing, rubbing, massaging, tasting, new smells, and bells and other sounding devices are all valuable sensory stimuli and can be used as reinforcers when the child shows pleasure in them. They can be combined with reflex-gross motor activities, patterning, follow hydrotherapy or, just be included periodically throughout the day. If aggressive sensory stimulation aggravates cerebral palsy or seizures, there are several alternatives. For example, fabrics with different textures can be placed gently on the infant's skin, a little perfume can be sprayed on nearby lamps, or a parent can sing softly. The following suggestions may prove most beneficial when designing this type of program for blind and blind, mentally retarded infants.

When a blind child functions at the level of a 4-month-old normal child, playing patty cake with him, letting him hold his bottle, placing little stocking mitts on his hands or putting a little honey or jelly on his fingers will draw his attention to his hands (Fraiberg, 1975). These activities help the child to sense the midline of his body and prepare him to use his hands in tandem. Later, he should be encouraged to reach out and touch toys, faces, and other safe objects. Parents should also bring objects to the child, place them in his hands, and name them carefully and repeatedly. These objects should include geometric solids such as cubes, cylinders, and cones, which will help the infant learn to identify and classify objects in the environment.

The infant can also be placed prone on the floor on a "texture pad"—which is made by sewing scraps of many types of fabric together and resembles a patchwork quilt. The pad can be made even more interesting by attaching bells and pieces of lace, knitting, rickrack, and elastic to the pad. Scents such as perfume, garlic, vanilla, and various other extracts can also be applied to the pad on occasion. Scents can also be added to the baby's bathwater. A "bathtime" basket may be arranged to be used when the baby is bathed. After exercising the baby in the bath, the parents can reach for items kept handy in a "bathtime" basket to brush and oil the child. After drying, the baby may be wrapped in fabrics of various textures.

Infants with some degree of responsiveness to light and color will benefit from appropriate visual stimulation. Rotating colored lamps used on Christmas trees or for outdoor lighting may provide some color interest if turned on for about five minutes in a darkened room. The light from penlights can be softened by placing a tissue over the tip. Colored tissue or cellophane will stimulate visual activity and may encourage some tracking and reaching. Caution should be exercised if the infant's condition includes seizures.

When the child functions at the 8- to 12-month level, he will benefit from a playpen, which not only is a space with recognizable perimeters but is an environment the infant can control. The playpen will be even more stimulating if a texture pad is placed on the bottom and sound toys are attached to a piece of elastic strung across the top. Toys such as measuring spoons, old keys on chains, and rattles can be attached to the sides with elastic. If larger toys, pillows, stuffed animals, cereal boxes, and paper are placed on the bottom, the infant will have obstacles to maneuver as well as maneuver around.

Because tactile development is limited until mobility skills are established (Cratty, 1971), blind children become more interested in touching and holding objects after they have begun to walk. Thus, healthy babies should be encouraged to crawl, walk barefoot, and pay close attention to the textures on floors and walls.

When the blind child functions at a 2½- to 3-year-old level, his tactile sensitivity can be enhanced as follows: have the child wash his hands in warm water and then guide his fingers over coarse and fine sandpaper, fabrics, and wallpaper samples. Discuss what he is feeling. (Older children can match sets of these items.) Let him feel warm and cold objects and learn the thermal and textural qualities of wood, plastic, and metal. These activities prepare him to learn the techniques that are essential to the mastery of braille or an Optacon reading device. Children who have the aptitude can be introduced to braille or the Optacon during their preschool years.

Language
Many blind and blind, mentally retarded children develop language skills extremely slowly—again, because mobility skills usually precede the development of language (Cratty, 1971; Umsted, 1975). Because language and eating involve much of the same musculature, Rogow (1973) urges parents of blind children to encourage oral activity of all types at an early age. Tactual stimulation of the child's oral cavity, throat, and sound-producing centers will aid the development of eating skills. (See *Project FAITH Curriculum for Infant Learning,* Mori & Olive, 1976, for additional suggestions.)

Parents can encourage and help the child develop language skills by telling him what is happening around him, identifying sounds in the environment, and naming objects he is handling at the time (Lowenfeld, 1964). Froyd (1973) encourages parents to use basic phrases with handicapped infants rather than meaningless noises, which he views as detrimental to learning. In the case of severe mental retardation, single, meaningful words must be repeated over and over again. Words such as mama, parts of the body, bottle, up, down, and milk, which represent objects or concepts that the child encounters frequently in the environment, are a good beginning.

Tape recordings of normal infant sounds can be played on a cassette recorder placed near the baby, and adults can imitate these sounds while playing with him. Immediate reward and parental enthusiasm will encourage the baby to respond. The "cough" game and parental imitation of the infant's sounds are most appropriate. Favorite lullabies, nursery rhymes, stories, proverbs, scriptures, numbers, and the words for colors can also be taped. Babies often respond to hearing their names called on the tapes. Parents should sing and repeat words the baby has heard on the tapes to make the sounds meaningful. Blos (1974) points out that blind children achieve a sense of orderliness when familiar words, stories, songs, and so forth are often repeated. This sense of orderliness is a result of memorization, which in turn is encouraged by the constancy of rhymes, fingerplay, games, and stories and other cultural representations.

Affect and independence
Researchers in the field of early childhood education for blind and visually handicapped, mentally retarded infants agree that these babies require immediate intervention in the affective domain of personality development (McGuire, 1971; Umsted, 1975). As Fraiberg, Smith, and Adelson (1969) point out: "No educational strategies can succeed if a baby has not found meaning in his world through his human partners and if he is not bound to this world through affectional ties to his parents."

Because bonding between infant and caretaker is so essential to the total development of the individual, parents should cuddle, coo to, and carry their blind infants as often as possible (Bobath, 1972). Blind African babies—who receive a normal amount of cultural stimulation and are carried often by their mothers—develop without the "blindisms" noted in Western cultures (Carolan, 1973). Fraiberg (1975) believes that a tactile dialogue, combined with abundant verbalization on the mother's part, is tremendously important; because the infant's responses are often infinitesimal, which does little to build parental confidence or acceptance, professional assistance may be required to establish this dialogue.

Lairy and Harrison-Covello (1973) found a positive correlation between maternal acceptance and the social, emotional, and cognitive functioning of visually handicapped children. A strategy must be found to help parents accept their blind babies as soon as possible (Umsted, 1975). Professionals can help the parents' acceptance by holding the baby, playing with him in a normal manner, pointing out his attractive features, and demonstrating obvious pleasure in and acceptance of him (Fraiberg, 1975).

Once bonding and acceptance is established, parents must be encouraged not to overprotect the baby. This can be most difficult. Teachers of the blind continually complain that many parents keep their blind children from developing normally because they fail to recognize their child's need for a strong self-concept and independence. McGuire and Meyers (1971) strongly urge that blind infants be given toys and an environment in which they can exert some control over objects as soon as possible. This is very important in the development of a strong self-image.

It is critical that the blind child be given training toward independence within the concept of normal developmental principles. Learning to dress himself, interact successfully with others, play, and develop toilet skills will assist the child in becoming independent. Feeding skills can be encouraged as soon as the baby sits by using finger foods (Fraiberg, Smith, & Adelson, 1969). Further suggestions for training in self-help skills are available in *The Project FAITH curriculum for infant learning* (Mori & Olive, 1976) and *The Project FAITH parent handbook* (Olive, 1976).

Young blind children need to play with other children. They are often isolated from others to a degree that later adds to their handicap (Bobath, 1972). Parents may have to make regular arrangements to provide socialization for their blind children. Pets are also helpful in developing affective responses when young blind children tend to be withdrawn.

Evaluation

The child's progress must be evaluated regularly to determine whether the program of intervention is effective and to improve the program if necessary. Many of the techniques and strategies described in this article have been used by staff members in Project FAITH, a demonstration project funded by the Bureau of Education for the Handicapped, U.S. Office of Education. Since October 1977, when the project was initiated, one blind and four blind, mentally retarded children ranging in age from 7 to 30 months have been referred to the project for services.

In Project FAITH, progress evaluations are essentially based on *The Project FAITH curriculum for infant learning* (Mori & Olive, 1976). Two evaluative tools are used. The first is "The Project FAITH developmental checklist," which corresponds in content and phases to the curriculum's general and specific goals and activities. Parents and staff complete the

checklist during the initial assessment phase and again six months after the child's program is initiated. The two sets of results are then compared. When this article was written, none of the children had been in the project for six months. The second instrument, the "Project FAITH worksheet," provides a more detailed analysis of the child's progress because it records the daily efforts made to accomplish specific goals outlined in each child's program. Thus, the staff has a written account of the specific objectives attempted and the number achieved. Many of the strategies described in this article are designed to attain specific behavioral goals. Although it would be imprudent to report specific numerical data at this stage, the preliminary findings are encouraging. The children in the program seem to be more responsive to stimulation, more alert, and behave more normally in important developmental areas than do other blind and blind, mentally retarded children.

Although this program emphasizes the need for intervention in early childhood, its ultimate goal is the greatest possible degree of normalization within adult society for blind and visually handicapped, mentally retarded individuals. Because early learning is generally easy learning and because early learning tends to persist, it is hoped that this program will provide an educational foundation for successful functioning in adulthood. Indeed, such a holistic educational design may eventually justify Wolfensberger's belief (1972) that "the facts justify the conclusion that the service system which will combine operant shaping techniques, activation, normalization, and intensive emphasis upon the young (age 0-6) impaired child will see successes of a degree beyond our power to conceptualize at this time."

References

Barry, M.A. (1973). How to play with your partially sighted preschool child: Suggestions for early sensory and educational activities. *New Outlook for the Blind, 12,* 457-467.

Bos, J.W. (1974). Rhymes, songs, records and stories: Language learning experiences for preschool blind children. *New Outlook for the Blind, 9,* 300-307.

Bobath, K. & Bobath, B. (1972). Cerebral palsy. In P.H. Pearson & C.E. Williams (eds.), *Physical therapy services in the developmental disabilities.* Springfield, IL: Charles C Thomas.

Bornstein, S. (1974). *Why severely impaired infants and their families need help. The*

earlier—the better. Boston: Boston Center for Blind Children.

Brazelton, T.B. (1975). Brazelton neonatal behavioral assessment. In B.Z. Friedlander, G.M. Sterritt, & G. Kirk (eds.), *Exceptional infant, Vol 3.* New York: Brunner/Mazel.

Brown M. (1977). Neurological basis for Ayre's theories of sensory integration. *Proceedings: Basic assessment and intervention techniques for deaf-blind and multihandicapped children.* California State Department of Education.

Burlingham, D. (1969). Review of Selma Fraiberg's "An educational program for blind infants." *Journal of Special Education, 3*(2), 141-142.

Carolan, R.H. (1973). Sensory stimulation: Two papers. *New Outlook for the Blind, 3,* 119-125.

Chase, J.B. (1975). Developmental assessment of handicapped infants and young children: With special attention to the visually impaired. *New Outlook for the Blind, 69*(8), 341-349.

Connelly, W. (1969). *Visually handicapped children: Birth to three years.* Ann Arbor: University of Michigan Press.

Cratty, B.J. (1971). *Movement and spatial awareness in blind children and youth.* Springfield, IL: Charles C Thomas.

Cratty B.J. (1972). The use of movement activities in the education of retarded children. In P.H. Pearson & C.E. Williams (eds.), *Physical therapy services in the developmental disabilities.* Springfield, IL: Charles C Thomas.

Dubose, R.F. (1976). Developmental needs in blind infants. *New Outlook for the Blind, 2,* 49-52.

Evans, B. & Summers, L. (1976). Normal and abnormal reflexes and their influences on motor behavior. *Presentations for Parents,* 40-56.

Fraiberg, S. (1975). Intervention in infancy: A program for blind infants. In B.Z. Friedlander, G.M. Sterritt, & G. Kirk (eds.), *Exceptional infant, Vol. 3.* New York: Brunner/Mazel.

Fraiberg, S., Smith, M., & Adelson, E. (1969). An educational program for blind infants. *Journal of Special Education, 3*(2), 121-139.

Froyd H.E. (1973). Counseling families of severely handicapped children. *New Outlook for the Blind, 67*(6), 251-257.

Gorham, K.A. (1975). A lost generation of parents. *Exceptional Children, 41,* 521-525.

Lairy, G.C. & Harrison-Covello, A. (1973). The blind child and his parents: Congenital visual defects and the repercussion of family attitudes on the early development of the child. *American Foundation for the Blind Research Bulletin, 25,* 1.

Leboyer, F. (1976). *Loving hands.* New York: Knopf.

Lowenfeld, B. (1964). *Our blind children:*

Growing and learning with them. Springfield, IL: Charles C Thomas.

Lowenfeld, B., Abel, G.L., & Hatlen, P.H. (1969). *Blind children learn to read.* Springfield, IL: Charles C Thomas.

McClennen, S. (1969). Teaching techniques for institutionalized blind retarded children. *New Outlook for the Blind,* **63**(10), 322-325.

McGuire, L.L. & Meyers, C.E. (1971). Early personality in the congenitally blind child. *New Outlook for the Blind,* **65**(5), 137-143.

Mainstreaming preschoolers: Children with visual handicaps. (1977). Belmont, MA: Contract Research Corp.

Mori, A.A. & Olive, J.E. (1976). *The Project FAITH curriculum for infant learning.* Las Vegas: University of Nevada.

Moss, J.W. & Mayer, D.L. (1975). Children with intellectual subnormality. In J.J. Gallager (ed.), *The application of child development research to exceptional children.* Reston, VA: Council for Exceptional Children.

Napier, G.D. (1974). *Handbook for teachers of the blind.* Louisville: American Printing House for the Blind.

Olive, J.E. (1976). *Project FAITH parent handbook for infant learning.* Las Vegas: University of Nevada.

Parad, H.J. (1975). Principles of crisis intervention. In H.J. Parad (ed.), *Emergency psychiatric care.* Bowie, MD: Charles Press.

Parker, A.L. (1971). Reinforcement: One teacher's experiences and experiments with multiply handicapped blind children. *New Outlook for the Blind,* **65**(3), 97-99.

Preschool learning activities for the visually impaired child: A guide for parents. (1972). Springfield: Illinois Instructional Materials Center.

Raynor, S. & Drouillard, R. (1975). *Get a wiggle on.* Mason, MI: Ingham Intermediate School District.

Raynor S. & Drouillard, R. (1975). *Move It.* Mason, MI: Ingham Intermediate School District.

Richards, S.S. & Briller, S. (1971). Learning from experience: A revisit to the children's corner. *New Outlook for the Blind,* **3**, 73-78.

Rogow, S.M. (1973). Speech development and the blind multi-impaired child. *Education of the Visually Handicapped,* **5**(4), 105-109.

Stockmeyer, S.A. (1972). A sensorimotor approach to treatment. In P.H. Pearson & C.E. Williams (eds.), *Physical therapy services in the developmental disabilities.* Springfield, IL.: Charles C Thomas.

Taylor, B.M. (1975). *Blind preschool: A manual for parents and educators.* Colorado Springs: SPED Publications.

Umsted, R.G. (1975). Children with visual handicaps. In J.J. Gallager (ed.), *The application of child development research to exceptional children.* Reston, VA: Council for Exceptional Children.

Voss, D.E. (1972). Proprioceptive neuromuscular facilitation: The PNF method. In P.H. Pearson & C.E. Williams (eds.), *Physical therapy services in the developmental disabilities.* Springfield, IL: Charles C Thomas.

Wardell, K.T. (1976). Parental assistance in orientation and mobility instruction. *New Outlook for the Blind,* **70**(8), 321-325.

Warnick, L. (1969). The effect upon a family of a child with a handicap. *New Outlook for the Blind,* **63**(10), 299-304.

Wolfensberger, W. (1972). *The Principle of normalization in human services.* Toronto: National Institute on Mental Retardation.

Allen A. Mori, Ph.D., director, Project FAITH and associate professor, Department of Special Education, University of Nevada, Las Vegas; Jane E. Olive, M.Ed., developmental specialist for Project FAITH.

The Rehabilitation Process for Persons Who Are Deaf and Blind

M. Nelipovich; L. Naegele

Abstract: The Rehabilitation Services Administration has identified deaf-blind persons as composing a priority population. The authors indicate the service delivery adaptations that professionals should consider when serving a deaf-blind client. The traditional vocational rehabilitation process is utilized as the service delivery model. Modifications of historical methods are suggested.

A host of factors affect the functional capacities of the deaf-blind person, among which are initial versus secondary impairments, complications (such as diabetes, epilepsy, or orthopedic impairments), severity of impairments, residual abilities, age at onset of disabilities, and overall social, economic, and developmental factors.

Examples of the variations found within the broad descriptor "deaf-blind" include: congenital deafness-blindness, i.e., individuals both aurally and visually impaired at birth; and adventitiously impaired individuals. This latter group is likely to exhibit even greater variation and includes persons "normal" at birth but who become aurally or visually impaired due to trauma (illness, accident, etc.). Also in this group are those persons congenitally aurally impaired and adventitiously visually impaired (as occurs with Usher's syndrome); and those congenitally visually impaired who become hearing impaired. It is important to be cognizant of the severity of the loss, the type of loss, and whether the individual was prelingually or adventitiously deafened. This variability strengthens the rationale for individualized services.

As much as possible, rehabilitation services should be adapted to fit the needs of the individual client. In 1974, Hammer proposed a new approach to rehabilitation services for deaf-blind persons. He suggested that the traditional approach to rehabilitation services based on a medical treatment model may not be suitable for many deaf-blind clients. He proposed a behavior model that would move an individual along a continuum toward various higher levels of independent functioning rather than toward a single job-related goal.

This discussion will focus upon the currently established sequence of services that exists within the state/federal system and the concerns that may be unique to the deaf-blind client. Due to its importance, its specialized modes of delivery, and its subjectivity to impairment when losses occur at an early age, the issue of communication deserves special discussion and will be the first topic to be dealt with.

Communication

Vernon (1973) reported that one-half of the deaf-blind population in this country are impaired as a consequence of Usher's syndrome. The rubella epidemic of 1963-1965 resulted in the birth of more aurally and visually handicapped children than were born during the Thalidomide disaster (Mindel & Vernon, 1971). Thousands of these children affected by rubella have hearing and vision impairments severe enough for them to be considered deaf-blind. Furthermore, of the 57 known forms of genetic deafness, 10 involve both hearing and vision (Mindel & Vernon, 1971).

This prelingually deaf group constitutes a substantial proportion of the deaf-blind population. While this by no means encompasses all deaf-blind persons, and while language difficulties are not necessarily present in a deaf-blind client, these figures indicate that there is likely to be a high proportion of clients who exhibit language difficulties due to early hearing impairment.

A prelingually deaf person with a severe neurosensory hearing loss is more than likely to suffer profound disruption in his or her communicative relations with the world. Despite a normal distribution of intelligence among deaf persons, over 30 percent are functionally illiterate (Vernon, 1970). Developing labels and symbols to organize the world and to eventually constitute "language" is a difficult, time-consuming task when auditory channels are eliminated or impaired. The deaf-blind or visually impaired child is even more likely to label and organize the world with idiosyncratic symbols that may not be common to the rest of the world. Therefore, it may be extremely difficult to decipher a deaf-blind person's representational system or to attempt to operate within it, since it may not correspond to the English language.

Rehabilitating the deaf-blind client necessitates dealing with each individual's unique and specialized communication needs. *Communication must be conducted at the client's level in a model that she or he prefers and is most comfortable with.* The rehabilitation service provider, therefore, must be cognizant of the developmental implications of deaf-blindness and must also be familiar with the wide range of language abilities and communication modes used by deaf-blind persons.

Table 1. Nineteen methods of communication identified by the literature as being developed for and used by the adult deaf-blind population (Yarnell, 1976).

1. The American One-Hand Manual Alphabet
2. The British Manual Alphabet
3. The Lorm Alphabet
4. The American Two-Hand Manual Alphabet
5. The International Morse Code
6. Braille Hand Speech
7. Sign Language (including American Sign Language and the recent array of manually coded sign systems)
8. The Alphabet Plate
9. The Alphabet Glove
10. The Talking Disc
11. Braille Alphabet Card
12. Cut-Out Letters
13. The Tadoma Method
14. Braille
15. Typing and Script Writing
16. The Tell-a-Touch Machine
17. The Tactaphone
18. Oral Speech
19. The International Standard Manual Alphabet (printing in the palm of the hand)

Table 1 indicates 19 different methods identified in the literature as being used by deaf-blind persons. This does not include any "home-made" system that might periodically surface. A 1976 study noted that many deaf-blind adults often know and can use more than one method, but all have methods that they strongly prefer and that best fit their own residual abilities and sensory preferences. The most preferred modes identified in the 1976 study were the American One-Hand Manual Alphabet (fingerspelling), American Sign Language (ASL), and printing in the palm of the hand (Yarnell, 1976).

It seems unreasonable to assume—particularly when considering the relatively low incidence of deaf-blindness—that all staff in all agencies should devote the time and energy needed to become fluent in a wide variety of methods as well as in what is essentially a foreign language (ASL). Many states have one or two specialists who can serve the deaf-blind client. For additional expertise, one could contact the regional representative from the Helen Keller National Center (HKNC) or one of the HKNC's approximately 20 affiliated agencies. Many state departments of vocational rehabilitation will have an Office for the Deaf and Hearing Impaired (ODHI), where interpreters may be found. If at all possible, evidence of skills should be required. Ideally, this would be certification through the Registry of Interpreters for the Deaf.

If an interpreter is to be used, both client and agency personnel should be or become familiar with how to properly work with an interpreter so as to avoid misunderstanding and/or placing undue pressure on the interpreter. Guidelines on interpreting and the proper use of interpreters can be obtained through Registry of Interpreters for the Deaf (R.I.D.), Inc., 814 Thayer Avenue, Silver Spring, Maryland 20910. An illustrated volume discussing the role and responsibilities of interpreting for deaf-blind persons, along with descriptions of many of the methods most commonly used, is available. It is appropriately entitled *Guidelines on Interpreting for Deaf-Blind Persons,* and can be obtained by writing to: Public Service Programs, Gallaudet College, Kendall Green, Washington, DC 20002.

Clients may sometimes have a preference regarding interpreters, and this should be honored if at all possible. The client and the agency also have the right to reject an interpreter (Rice & Simmons, 1974).

A person skilled in communication should be with the deaf-blind individual throughout each phase of the rehabilitation process rather than just at selected times. The literature on rehabilitation services for the deaf is replete with examples of difficulties encountered by the deaf individual during the rehabilitation process. Boyd and Boros (1975) cite the following as major contributors to deficits in service delivery to hearing impaired persons:

1. Serious communication problems
   a. Hearing
   b. Speaking
   c. Reading and writing
2. Lack of sophistication
   a. Confusion over bureaucratic complexities
   b. Ignorance of professional role behavior
   c. Inadequate formal education
3. Fear of exploitation by hearing persons
4. Self-segregation (Sussman & Stewart, 1971)
5. Over-dependency on:
   a. Helpers (e.g., interpreters, etc.)
   b. Relatives
   c. Deaf leaders
6. Low economic status
7. Under-aspiring in:
   a. Vocational areas (Vernon, 1970)
   b. Educational areas (Vernon, 1970)
   c. Social spheres

Casefinding and referral

Outreach and referral may require special efforts on the part of the rehabilitation agency. The agency should develop rapport with schools, both residential and day, to identify children needing services as early as possible. Traditionally, educational and rehabilitation programs for deaf-blind persons have been conducted by programs serving visually impaired persons. This continues to be true for the most part. Coordination between Individualized Education Programs (IEPs) and Individualized Written Rehabilitation Programs (IWRPs) is essential and is required by the 1978 amendments of the 1973 Rehabilitation Act.

Other sources of referral are state hospitals, mental health centers, nursing homes, audiologists, otologists, speech pathologists, ophthalmologists, optometrists, hearing-aid dealers, opticians, speech and hearing centers, low-vision centers, rehabilitation centers, welfare agencies, and the Social Security Administration. National, state, and local organizations for the deaf or blind should also be explored.

It must be remembered that attempts to contact deaf-blind persons through the usual media may prove unsuccessful. For example, radio, television, newspapers, magazines, workshops, etc., may not be readily accessible to the deaf-blind persons; therefore, extra effort is necessary.

Personal contacts and home visits are to be encouraged.

Intake

Intake is a crucial point in the rehabilitation process. One of the first tasks of the intake interview is the development of understanding and confidence between the client and the case manager (Bitter, 1979). The first few minutes of the initial contact can set the tone for mutual understanding and a positive working atmosphere that will permeate later dealings (Bettica, 1979). So, meaningful communication is to be striven for from the outset. To do this requires an atmosphere of trust and a correction of distortion in communication through feedback (Bitter, 1979).

Accurate communication is particularly important at this point since a good deal of fairly critical information needs to be gathered and discussed. Counselor/case manager roles need to be explained; services and steps in the rehabilitation process need to be delineated; and the IWRP client's rights and responsibilities, the agency's responsibilities, functions and limits, as well as the appeal process, should be understood by the client (Lafitte, 1979).

Communication and content level should be as appropriate as possible. If information is available before the client arrives regarding language levels and preferred method(s) of communication, advance plans can be made. Having a skilled communicator or interpreter, or necessary specialized equipment ready, is a necessity.

There is often a tendency to believe, especially if the client's visual or auditory impairment is not total or profound, that notewriting or lipreading will be sufficient. This is a misconception, and skills in those areas should not be assumed. Unless the client states that this is his or her preferred method of communicating, depending solely upon written or spoken communication is to be avoided. Other factors, such as seating, lighting, and distance from counselor to client, are of similar importance. The counselor or intake person should take the time to assess the client carefully, and lengthy explanations due to lack of sophistication are highly likely (Boyd & Boros, 1975). Due to this, time should be extended and scheduled for as much as twice the time used for normal verbal interviews. If this initial contact is hurried, tense, or fraught with confusion, frustration, and misconceptions, there is a risk that the client may be lost at this early stage.

The amount of information and the depth of explanation should be appropriate to the client's level of understanding. However, it should be remembered that an individual's communication preference may reveal little about his or her other potentials and abilities (Rice & Simons, 1974). Abilities such as facility with the English language, speech/speechreading, or braille reading and writing, are highly dependent upon such factors as age of onset of the disability and previous training. They do not indicate or negate intelligence. At the termination of the initial contact, specific instructions regarding the next scheduled appointment(s) should be given and checked for understanding. Usually, having dates, places, times, contact persons, etc., in some form that the client can take along (written, large print, brailled, etc.) is helpful and is recommended.

Diagnosis

Determining rehabilitation program eligibility and subsequent services is the responsibility of the rehabilitation counselor in the federal/state program. A preliminary diagnostic study is generally conducted during the application phase of the rehabilitation process in order to determine the existence and extent of the disabling condition(s) that will constitute a substantial barrier to employment.

In all cases, diagnosis includes a general medical examination. This should include both a medical history and a conventional anatomical and pathological examination. Minimally, the medical history should provide the client's chief complaint, a history of past or present illnesses, a family history, the individual's habits, a vocational history, a psychosocial history, and a systemic review (Bitter, 1979).

However, the general medical examination does not include detailed information regarding an individual's auditory and visual functioning. The inappropriate use of the term "deaf-blind" might handicap the client more by creating an inappropriate image in the mind's eye of a potential employer or potential supervisor. Only a very small percentage of so-called "deaf-blind" individuals are, in fact, totally deaf or totally blind (Monk, 1976). A description of hearing and vision impairment in more precise, operational terms will probably be more meaningful to all concerned.

Ophthalmological and optometric examinations, plus audiological and otological evaluations, should be obtained for every client and be the source of evidence to substantiate the vision and hearing impairments.

These diagnostic scores will, among other things, give valuable insight into an individual's sensory strengths and preferences and will largely determine whether he or she will be considered a hearing and visually impaired person ("deaf-blind," with deafness being the predominant disabling condition) or visually and hearing impaired ("blind-deaf") person. This information will then be valuable in determining the appropriateness of various assistive devices, services, and training. The feasibility of restorative surgery to improve or retain either sight or hearing should be determined at this point and recommendations made regarding the appropriateness of such action.

It is recommended that the previously mentioned ophthalmological/otological reports include the following information (Lafitte, 1979):
• the anatomical condition of the eyes and ears;
• a quantitative estimate of the degree of vision/hearing loss;
• presence or absence of other symptoms (such as blood clots, high tonometry readings, vertigo tinnitus, etc.); and
• etiology, prognosis, and recommendations for medical treatment or surgery and evaluation for assistive devices (such as glasses, hearing aids, or low-vision aids).

Audiological evaluations should be done by an audiologist certified and/or licensed in accordance with the state laws and regulations. This report should include a description of the extent and type of loss as well. Furthermore, if a recommendation for amplification is made, the following information should be included: the ear to be fitted, type of aid, specific characteristics of the aid vis-à-vis the client's needs, length of trial period, and an indication that an orientation to the aid was given. The client's reactions to the aid should also be noted. Impedance audiometry and speech audiometry outcomes should be recorded in the report as well (Lafitte, 1979).

The parallel to the hearing aid evaluation is the low vision assessment. Although certification and/or licenses do not as yet exist for this specialty, most larger cities will have at least one or two persons qualified to perform such an evaluation. Some optometrists and ophthalmologists are trained in low vision assessment. The low vision specialist should be recommended by a local agency that deals largely with visually impaired persons.

The report should include information similar to that found in an audiological evaluation for devices (type of devices, possibility of benefits from magnification, specific characteristics of the devices suggested as related to the client's needs, indication of orientation to the aids, and so on). Again, accurate information regarding the client's current and potential auditory and visual functioning is a necessity.

Evaluation

In the event that rehabilitation potential cannot be immediately determined but disabling condition(s) have been established, the public program provides for an extended evaluation period not exceeding 18 months (Bitter, 1979). Most aurally and visually impaired clients can benefit from extended services (Rice & Simmons, 1974). In addition to the medical evaluations, biographical information should be collected so as to provide a global profile from which hypotheses about skills, abilities, and adjustments may be developed (Watson, 1979).

Evaluations or specific skills and aptitude areas should be as comprehensive as possible to provide a basis for future planning aimed at developing all of a person's assets. However, few of the existing tools for evaluation, particularly the psychometric measures of personality and interests, can be used with any confidence when assessing severely handicapped persons (Watson, 1979). Additionally, few general rehabilitation counselors, psychologists, or evaluators have the knowledge, skill, or experience to appropriately assess the deaf-blind individual. Misdiagnosis, particularly of mental retardation or mental illness, is highly likely and often occurs when standard measures are administered and interpreted by professionals without sufficient knowledge of and exposure to the implications of the disabilities involved. Selectivity should be exercised when determining who will conduct and interpret the psychometric testing, as well as in accepting previous test results when the administrator, methods, and adaptations are unknown.

Work samples and situational assessments offer significant advantages over traditional psychometric tests (Watson, 1979). They have considerable face validity and allow the client to work with tools and materials identical to those found in an actual job setting in a realistic manner. Not only are work samples based on performance rather than on verbal responses, they also give valuable information about fine and gross dexterity and motor coordination and indicate physical tolerance and work behaviors. They also provide the client with first-hand experience with various tasks and working environments.

Watson (1979) proposes a model for the vocational evaluation of deaf clients that follows a sequential pattern described by Nadolsky (1971). The general sequence is portrayed as a continuous process leading from the collection of biographical data to placement and/or improved adjustment. In addition to the regular components of psychological tests, work samples, situational try-outs, counseling, etc., a strong communication base and concurrent social and work adjustment services are present from the initial stage. The presence of these additional services provides a "total adjustment environment" within which a client can be assessed and eventually rehabilitated. This is suggested because the primary difficulties encountered in the evaluation and adjustment of such severely disabled clients appear to be deficient social and emotional functioning that "stultifies achievement and precludes occupational attainment" (Watson, 1979). Since deficits in personal or social areas are likely to exist in the prelingually deaf-blind client, an environment that concurrently assesses and fosters client adjustment and functioning may help alleviate some of the complicating factors that can interfere with valid vocational functioning.

For example, psychometric and single-work-sample assessments might indicate dubious vocational potential. However, ongoing evaluation given as support services and training are implemented may provide behavioral evidence of more potential than was initially indicated. This type of evaluation setting is suggested for clients who demonstrate the aforementioned deficits or are highly likely to possess them. A total adjustment environment may be appropriate for other aspects of assessment as well, since strengths and deficits may exist in a number of areas, several of which are crucial to independent functioning (i.e., activities of daily living, use of leisure time, social skills, orientation and mobility).

It should be remembered that, regardless of the skill of the individuals administering most tests and evaluations, the results should not be considered precise. The lack of standardized, normed, and validated evaluation instruments for deaf-blind persons (with the possible exception of some work-sample systems) makes precise statements nearly impossible. The results, coupled with the evaluator's observations and impressions, can only serve as general indicators of current and potential functioning upon which future planning can be based.

The process is likely to be more time-consuming and expensive due to the use of specialized equipment, extended staff time, and laborious communication. It may well also be confusing because of uneven test results, widely varying language levels, knowledge gaps, and other extreme variations from client to client. What seems to be needed is a specialist in deaf-blind rehabilitation equivalent to rehabilitation counselors for the blind or deaf.

Eligibility

Eligibility is, of course, a crucial determination. Deafness-blindness is considered by RSA regulations as a severe disability, and hence the deaf-blind individual is likely to be determined eligible if the evaluations indicate vocational potential.

The difficulty here may be with the focus on vocational potential and case closure. If the evaluation phase is not conducted by persons with a thorough knowledge of deafness-blindness and its implications (and sometimes even if it is), there may be serious questions regarding the individual's potential, and the client may be turned down by the agency as having no identifiable vocational goal (Hammer, 1974). Clearly, no client should be refused services without the opportunity to link up with person(s) knowledgeable in the area of deafness-blindness. Additionally, there may be a need to reevaluate traditional vocational rehabilitation (VR) criteria. Permanent case closure may in fact not be the end goal for some of these clients. The multiply handicapped, deaf-blind individual may never achieve independence without requiring extended support services.

This underscores the need for as accurate an assessment as possible and some amendments in the end goals of the rehabilitation process, such as reduction in dependence as opposed to competitive employment or independent living. The deaf-blind client may not have a clear understanding of what the functions of the VR agency are. The client may be unaware of the services he or she is entitled to and will or will not receive if turned down by the agency. These should be explained as fully as possible at various points during the process.

Individualized Written Rehabilitation Program (IWRP)

After the evaluation has identified the client's needs, strengths, deficits, and interests, concrete planning can begin. The IWRP is to be jointly developed by the disabled person and the counselor. If the client cannot be actively involved, it is done through a parent, guardian, or appropriate advocate. The IWRP includes: 1) the basis for eligibility or extended evaluation; 2) long-range employment goals; 3) intermediate rehabilitation objectives; 4) identification of services needed to achieve the end goal(s); 5) expected dates for beginning and ending the detailed services; and 6) a schedule for evaluating progress in the attainment of goals and objectives (Department of Health, Education and Welfare, 1974). Communication skills are important because the IWRP requires that the client be involved and understand as fully as possible the policies, procedures, and responsibilities of all involved.

Since recent changes have begun to emphasize the need for all types of services necessary for complete rehabilitation (Hicks, 1978), VR should focus on independence-oriented goals as well as on vocational goals for the deaf-blind client. The IWRP should reflect this.

Once again, developing the IWRP and discussing it with the client may be a laborious and time-consuming process. Depending upon the knowledge of the individual involved, very fundamental issues and vocabulary may require explanation. Although potentially time-consuming, as much explanation as can be done should be done. Not only is this required, but it may significantly aid in a client being involved with and supportive of his or her programming and services.

Adjustment training

In rehabilitation, training refers to a broad range of learning opportunities and experiences that will help the client progress to the employment goal of the IWRP (Bitter, 1979). Since adequate psychological and interpersonal functioning can be considered a prerequisite to the maintenance of employment, personal adjustment services play an important role in the rehabilitation of many disabled clients. Key problems for rehabilitation clients include inability to communicate in a facilitative manner, ineffective behaviors in important life situations, low desire for achievement, expectation of external control over one's fate, ineffective problem-solving and goal-setting skills, and inability to use community resources (Rubin & Roessler, 1978).

Personal-adjustment services refer to the development of habits and attitudes related to adjustment in the world of work (Bitter, 1979). These skills could be broadly referred to as prevocational skills. This training can be delivered in a variety of settings—hospitals, rehabilitation facilities, and rehabilitation field offices within the client's community (Rubin & Roessler, 1978). It is naturally imperative that the service providers to whom the deaf-blind client is referred for training possess the appropriate expertise and skills for working effectively with this select population.

Vocational training refers to the development of specific job skills (Bitter, 1979). It is important that no skill be arbitrarily or firmly decided upon until a complete, professional evaluation is conducted. The client's skills, abilities, and functional capacities as well as the demands of potential jobs must be considered to determine an appropriate match (Rubin & Roessler, 1978). Evaluators as well as counselors and trainers should therefore be aware of the potential employment market for the deaf-blind person so as to provide appropriate training.

Vocational training may take place in a rehabilitation facility, sheltered workshop, vocational school, or other academic setting. One should be sure, particularly in academic settings, that support services are available (readers, notetakers, etc.).

Counseling

Bitter (1979) described rehabilitation counseling as a process involving a counselor and a client to help the client make effective use of personal and environmental resources for the best possible vocational, personal and social adjustment. In this respect, a client is viewed holistically; that is, he or she is not merely divided into abstract parts, such as physical, mental, social, and economic.

The counselor needs to be sensitive to the wide range of ramifications related to deafness-blindness. This aspect of rehabilitation is especially important with a client who is facing the recent or progressive loss of an additional sense, particularly when the individual is highly dependent upon that sense, as would occur in cases such as those with Usher's syndrome. Certainly, the emotional and behavioral implications of coping with such a secondary loss cannot be underestimated. Hammer (1979) states that, if an individual does *not* exhibit stressful behavior, there is a need to be concerned about the person's mental health, for "to act normal in such an abnormal situation is to deny the impact of the situation."

The situation should certainly not be ignored and warrants exploration and discussion. The counselor may choose to address this need or to refer the client to psychological services, depending on the severity of the emotional responses the client exhibits. The need for counseling may further extend to parents and family members so they as well can provide encouragement, understanding, and a supportive environment.

High-quality communication is a must. Ideally, especially within the counseling relationship, the counselor should possess the necessary communication skills. If this is not possible, the use of a skilled interpreter is a must. Counseling the severely multiply handicapped person may require a certain level of time and patience that not all counselors possess.

Placement

Ever since 1920, placement has been regarded as the culminating service, the goal of the entire vocational rehabilitation process (Wright, 1980). One of the most substantial contributions a rehabilitation counselor can make, which affects the client's overall mental and physical adjustment, is the placement of the individual in a job that is well suited to his or her abilities and interests (Cull & Hardy, 1972). Some agencies have a professional placement specialist who relieves the counselor at this stage of the rehabilitation process. Bitter (1979) highlighted five rehabilitation-counselor role orientations to placement:

1. *Arranger.* The arranger-oriented counselor considers the placement function to be an opportunity to refer the client to others who can put him or her in contact with suitable employment. This placement activity consists of coordinating, conferring, and cooperating with other agencies or persons.

2. *Agent.* The agent-oriented counselor considers placement function to be a job of selling the client to prospective employers.

3. *Instructors.* The instructor-oriented counselor attempts to teach the client behaviors that will help him or her obtain a job.

4. *Guide.* The guide-oriented counselor views himself as an information resource for the client.

5. *Therapist.* The therapeutic counselor views the placement function as assisting the client to better attain self-understanding. The therapeutic counselor reasons that such understanding will help the client match his or her capacities and limitations to employment opportunities.

The level of skills of the individual deaf-blind client will largely dictate which of these approaches will be most appropriate. The complexities of deafness-blindness may require the professional to utilize several of these strategies. Whichever technique is used, the rehabilitation counselor or placement specialist must be concerned with both client and employer preparation.

Follow-up

Gains made in rehabilitation training and placement of the client must be reinforced as clients make the transition to full-time employment. Awareness of the importance of this aspect of the process is imperative for the rehabilitation professional. George Nelson Wright (1980) described the follow-up service as

> supportive assistance during the initial stages of job placement to evaluate the adequacy of rehabilitation services, to ascertain the client's need for further services, to determine whether job placement is satisfactory, to decide when the case can be closed, and to provide closure data.

It is highly likely that the deaf-blind client will require closer, more frequent follow-ups. This will likely be the case in terms of independent functioning as well as employment.

Follow-up services could indicate further adjustment services, immediate intervention if difficulties surface, employment maintenance, employer assistance, and accountability data for the rehabilitation agency. Federal regulations indicate that state agency cases should not be closed for at least 60 days after the client has been on the job. Status 31, post-employment services, allows VR cases to remain open and services to continue for a longer period of time (12 months).

Service delivery

Historically, blindness has always been regarded as the most severe disabling condition and, as a result, the deaf and blind person was traditionally served by agencies whose focal population was blind persons. This may not be the most effective form of service delivery. In the states that have a general agency and an agency serving blind persons, who should carry the case is still often in question. Perhaps the primary disabling condition could determine this issue. But again, who determines this needs to be clarified. Coordination between services to the deaf and services to the blind for jointly handling all initial referrals and screening of deaf-blind clients, and thereafter offering transfer to an appropriate case manager, might be an initial step.

The obvious danger of not having an effective referral and case-management system is that the deaf-blind person may receive quasi-professional services. A further solution would be to identify someone as the coordinator of services to the deaf-blind population in each state to insure that the deaf-blind consumer receives all available services.

Conclusion
This article has attempted to highlight the nuances of deaf-blindness and the rehabilitation process. Once case finding develops a more positive posture, vocational rehabilitation will be providing services to more of these individuals. The uniqueness of this handicap will require many professionals to seek more knowledge and understanding in communications, evaluation, placement and other areas in the rehabilitation process.

References
Barcomb, D. (1976). Vocational needs of the deaf-blind. *Proceedings of the OCPRWAD Spring Conference on Deaf-Blind*. Columbus, OH: Madison County Board of Education.

Bettica, L. (1979) Counseling the Usher's syndrome deaf-blind individuals. *Journal of Rehabilitation of the Deaf, 12, 4*.

Bitter, J.J. (1979). *Introductions to vocational rehabilitations*. St. Louis, MO: C.V. Mosby.

Boyd, D. & Boros, A. (1975). Bridging the gap with deaf paraprofessionals. *Journal of Rehabilitation of the Deaf, 8, 4*.

English, L. (1978) (ed.). Usher's syndrome, the personal, social and emotional implications. *American Annals of the Deaf, 123, 3*.

Hammer, E. (1974). Needs of deaf-blind persons. *Journal of Rehabilitation of the Deaf, 8, 1*.

Hicks, D. (1974). Usher's syndrome: Programmatic considerations. *American Annals of the Deaf, 8, 1*.

Lafitte, J. (1979). *A model state plan for the vocational rehabilitation of the deaf*. Richmond, VA: Virginia Department of Rehabilitative Services.

Mindel, E.D. & Vernon, M. (1971). *They grow in silence*. Silver Spring, MD: National Association of the Deaf.

Monk, G. (1976). Regional overview of services to deaf-blind children. *Proceedings of the OCPRWAD Spring Conference on Deaf-Blind*. Columbus, OH: Madison County Board of Education.

O'Rourke, T.J. (1973). *A basic course in manual communication*. Silver Springs, MD: National Association of the Deaf.

Rice, B.D. & Simmons, G. (1974). *Serving deaf rehabilitation clients: Fundamentals of communication for the general counselor*. Hot Springs, AR: University of Arkansas, Arkansas Rehabilitation Research and Training Center and Hot Springs Rehabilitation Center.

Rubin, S.E. & Roessler, R.T. (1978). *Foundations of the vocational rehabilitation process*. Baltimore: University Park Press.

Schein, J. (1973). Model state plan for vocational rehabilitation of deaf clients. *Journal of Rehabilitation of the Deaf*. Monograph No. 3

Vernon, M. (1969). Usher's syndrome: Deafness and progressive blindness; clinical cases, preventive theory and literature survey. *Journal of Chronic Diseases, 22*.

Vernon, M. (1970). Potential achievement and rehabilitation of the deaf population. *Rehabilitation Literature, 13, 9*.

Vernon, M. (1973). Overview of Usher's syndrome: Congenital deafness and progressive loss of vision. *Proceedings of Usher's Syndrome Conference*. Washington, DC: Gallaudet College.

Watson, D. (1973). Guidelines for the psychological and vocational assessments of deaf rehabilitation clients. *Journal of Rehabilitation of the Deaf, 13, 1*.

Wright, G.N. (1980). *Total rehabilitation*, Boston: Little, Brown.

Wyrick, D. (1979). Rehabilitation of deaf-blind adults: The role of the comprehensive vocational rehabilitation adjustment training center. *Journal of Rehabilitation of the Deaf, 12, 4*.

Yarnell, G. (1976). Communication needs of the deaf-blind. Proceedings of the OCPRWAD Conference on Deaf-Blind. Columbus, OH: Madison County Board of Education.

Michael Nelipovich, Ph.D., coordinator, Blind and Visually Impaired Services, Department of Health and Social Services, Madison, WI; Lois Naegele, M.A., Counselor, Hearing Impaired Program, Anna Mental Health and Development Center, Anna, IL.

EXPRESSIONS

Visually handicapped individuals with multiple disabilities exert increased control over events as they become effective communicators.
The two articles which follow provide evidence that a meaningful environment is the key to the development of a functional language system.

Training Pragmatic Language Skills Through Alternate Strategies with a Blind Multiply Handicapped Child

C.J. Evans; C.J. Johnson

Abstract: A blind multiply handicapped preschool child was taught to respond appropriately to two adjacency pair types. *Where Question - Answer* and *Comment - Acknowledgement*. Training involved teaching manual searching behavior as an alternate strategy for visual searching in response to "where" questions. Echolalic responses to comments initially served only a turn-taking function but, through explicit modification, gradually evolved into more appropriate and communicative responses. The blind child's appropriate responses to trained adjacency pair types increased significantly over the 14-week treatment period. The success of this program augers well for future efforts to develop communication-based interventions that incorporate the alternate language acquisition strategies available to blind children.

Vision plays an important role in normal language development through the establishment of communicative interaction at an early age. Visual cues are necessary for establishing mutual reference (Landau, 1983; Wills, 1979), developing a gesture system that facilitates comprehension and use of linguistic structures (Wood, 1981; Clark & Sengul, 1978), and regulating communicative interactions (McGurk, 1983; Mulford, 1983).

Vision also facilitates development of the cognitive foundations for language (Cromer, 1973; Piaget & Inhelder, 1969). Through observation and interaction with the environment, sighted children learn about the world. Word meanings are gradually acquired by pairing the language that is heard with events and objects observed in the environment (Nelson, 1978).

The inability to see may force blind children to acquire communicative skills and language content via different routes than those available to sighted children. Garman (1983) hypothesizes:

Given intact vision, certain strategies will

This article is based on a research project completed by the first author in partial fulfillment of the requirements for the Master of Clinical Science degree in Communicative Disorders at the University of Western Ontario. Portions of this article were presented at the 1985 annual meeting of the Ontario Speech and Hearing Association in Toronto.

regularly be employed en route to certain language abilities, but also without this faculty certain alternative [and ultimately specifiable] strategies are available, to achieve the same end.

Two possible alternative language acquisition strategies available to blind children are the use of echolalia to maintain communicative interactions and the use of manual searching to learn about the environment. Blind children may acquire language skills without associating them with the context in which they occur. As a result, blind children may rely heavily on the strategy of using echolalia, either immediate or delayed, in "unanalyzed chunks" to acquire language (Andersen, Dunlea, & Kekelis, 1984). Echolalic utterances in the language of blind children have been observed to maintain social contact and interaction, to function as requests, to provide self-direction, and to occur in word-play routines (Ford, 1984; Kitzinger, 1984). Echolalia, thus, may represent a unique, but important, language acquisition strategy (Fay, 1973; Schuler, 1979; Prizant & Duchan, 1981; Prizant, 1982) for some handicapped learners, including blind children.

Manual searching provides the blind child with valuable information about the environment and, in turn, enables them to communicate this knowledge. Manual searching may function as an alternative

strategy for the visual searching and observation that facilitates conceptual development in sighted children (Cromer, 1983).

The designation of echolalia and manual searching as possible alternative language acquisition strategies is supported by empirical descriptions of the behaviors of blind children. Echolalia is a frequently reported characteristic of the language of blind children (Andersen, *et al.*, 1984; Ford, 1984; Urwin, 1984a). Blind children use manual searching to a greater extent than do their sighted peers (Fraiberg, 1977).

Training studies provide stronger support for the designation of echolalia and manual searching as alternative language acquisition strategies. If training based on these alternative strategies facilitates language skill, it could be argued that these strategies are sufficient, in context, to enhance linguistic growth.

This case study was initiated in order to determine whether training that considered two alternative language acquisition strategies, echolalia and manual searching, would facilitate development of a blind child's pragmatic language skills, specifically the skill of appropriate responding to adjacency pairs. Clark and Clark (1977) define an adjacency pair as "a pair of utterances from two speakers in which the first elicits the second, as in a question-answer or greeting-greeting sequence." The use of adjacency pairs requires the ability to communicate and to grasp language content, two areas of linguistic skill that are problematic for blind children (Andersen, *et al.*, 1984). Nieuwesteeg (1981) and Ford (1984) found that blind children were slower to acquire appropriate responses to adjacency pairs, suggesting that direct teaching might enhance these skills.

Method

Subject

The subject, Peter, three years old, and six months old at the initiation of the study, is congenitally blind due to optic atrophy. Delays in both gross and fine motor development were shown in his inability to walk unaided and his limited manual strength and dexterity, characteristics frequently associated with congenital blindness (Fraiberg, 1977; Urwin, 1984b). Multiply handicapped blind children, such as Peter, are at greater risk for language impairment than blind children without associated handicaps (Elstner, 1983) and, therefore, are especially appropriate as subjects in evaluations of the

Table 1. Subject characteristics: Pre- and post-treatment measures.

Measure	Pre-treatment	Post-treatment
Chronological age	42 months	46 months
Receptive-expressive language assessment[a]		
Receptive language age	34 months	47 months
Expressive language age	42 months	51 monhts
Spontaneous language sample measures		
Mean length of utterance (MLU)[b]	2.92 morphemes	3.77 morphemes
Predicted CA based on MLU[c]	27-40 months	32-48 months
Initiations/total utterances[d]	16%	27%
Echolalic/total utterances	16%	17%
Mitigated/echolalic utterances	14%	23%
Manual searching (# times/3 baselines)	35	68
Appropriate adjacency pair responses	45/108 = 42%	71/108 = 66%
*Where Question - Answer	7/18 = 39%	11/18 = 61%
*Comment - Acknowledgement	3/18 = 17%	14/18 = 78%
Yes/No Question - Answer	6/18 = 33%	7/18 = 39%
What Question - Answer	11/18 = 61%	13/18 = 72%
Offer - Acceptance/Rejection	6/18 = 33%	11/18 = 61%
Command - Grant/Denial	12/18 = 67%	15/18 = 83%

*Trained adjacency pair

[a](Anderson & Smith, 1979); [b](Brown, 1973); [c](Miller, 1981); [d](Fey, 1986)

practical significance of a language training procedure.

Peter demonstrated delays in both his gross and fine motor development, characteristics that are frequently associated with congenital blindness (Fraiberg, 1977; Urwin, 1984b). Neurological examination at 14 months revealed hypotonicity, with no rigidity or spasticity, and weakness in all extremities. Peter was not walking unaided or completely toilet trained during the investigation period. Peter's hand skills were limited; his fingers and hands lacked strength; and he was unable to coordinate bilateral activities. Proprioceptive and vestibular functioning were also impaired; Peter was not aware of his center of balance while walking with support. He experienced delays in comprehension of basic concepts, a relative strength in memory skills, and a high degree of variability. Multiply handicapped blind children, such as Peter, are at greater risk of language impairment than blind children without associated handicaps.

Pre-treatment language skills
Peter's language skills were formally assessed at the initiation of the study through administration of the *Receptive Expressive Language Assessment* (Anderson & Smith, 1979). Peter's expressive language age score of 42 months (CA = 42 months) was higher than his receptive score of 34 months, suggesting that some of his verbalizations were not meaningful to him. Peter exhibited particular difficulties on test items which required the receptive knowledge of familiar object names and simple prepositions.

After Peter had interacted with the experimenter on several occasions, a spontaneous language sample was videotaped to estimate aspects of his pretreatment conversational proficiency. Results of relevant initial language sample measures are shown in Table 1.

As language is an interaction of form, content, and use (Bloom & Lahey, 1978), Peter's initial language competence revealed a pattern often seen in blind children (Andersen, *et al.*, 1984): relatively strong expressive syntax skills (form), but relatively weak vocabulary and conceptual skills (content), coupled with problems in appropriate conversational interaction (use).

Materials
Examples of the six adjacency pairs selected for study are listed in Table 2. In

Table 2. Adjacency pair types and examples.

*Where Question-Answer
  Example: E:"Where is the ball?"
         S:"Under the table."
*Comment - Acknowledgement
  Example: E:"This doll is mine."
         S:"No, it's mine."
Yes/No Question-Answer
  Example: E:"Did you have a nap today?"
         S-(shakes head)
What Question-Answer
  Example: E:"What do I have?"
         S:"A bell"
Offer - Acceptance/Rejection
  Example: E:"Let's play with the cars."
         S:"No, the farm."
Command - Grant/Denial
  Example: E:"Put the instruments in the box."
         S:"OK" (puts instruments in box)

*Trained adjacency pair

order to provide a comprehensive sampling of Peter's responses to these adjacency pairs, three different assessment lists were developed. Each list consists of a total of 36 elicitation sentences, six sentences for each of the six adjacency pairs. All object names used in the elicitation sentences were familiar to Peter. An attempt was made to equate vocabulary level and syntactic structure across the three elicitation lists.

Procedure
Initial baseline data were collected over three sessions during a one-week period (Figure 1). The three adjacency pair elicitation lists were randomly matched to the three initial baselines.

Each baseline session lasted approximately 20-25 minutes and was videotaped. Within a play situation, the experimenter took advantage of naturally occurring opportunities to present adjacency pair elicitation sentences from the assessment list.

The videotape of each baseline session was transcribed and analyzed to determine Peter's responses in the target adjacency pairs. Responses were initially classified as appropriate or inappropriate. Appropriate responses were further sub-classified as verbal or nonverbal. Inappropriate responses were sub-classified as either (a) incorrect, (b) echolalic, (c) verbal-nonverbal inconsistency, (d) indiscriminate affirmative, or (e) no response. (The adjacency pair elicitation lists and definitions for sub-classifications are available upon request from the authors.)

The treatment period lasted 14 weeks and included 36 sessions, each approximately 30 minutes in length. Single baseline sessions were conducted at nine-session intervals throughout the treatment phase to monitor changes in Peter's performance. Final baseline data were collected over three sessions during a one-week period (Figure 1). Baseline sessions during the treatment and final assessment phases were conducted and analyzed in the same manner as were the initial baselines.

Two adjacency pair types, *Where Question-Answer* and *Comment-Acknowledgement,* were targetted in the intervention program. *Where Question-Answer* was trained in order to facilitate the development of manual searching behavior, which Peter rarely performed. The *Comment-Acknowledgement* adjacency pair initially elicited echolalic responses from Peter, suggesting that he was aware of conversational turn-taking rules but unable to generate an appropriate response. This adjacency pair was included in the training

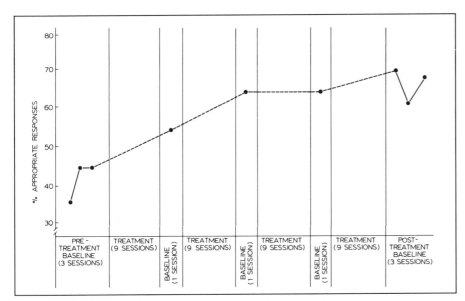

Figure 1. Time frame for baseline and treatment of phases of the study, showing the percentage of appropriate responses to all adjacency pairs as a function of treatment time.

procedure to reduce indirectly echolalia by providing Peter with alternative, more appropriate responses.

To teach manual searching responses, we used two types of games. In the hide-seek game, Peter was taught to search for a desired object in a variety of hiding places. In the object discrimination game, Peter learned to feel an array of objects in order to find one specified by the experimenter. Verbal encouragement and physical guidance were used initially but were faded as Peter's skill and independence in manual search improved. The level of difficulty of the teaching tasks was systematically increased by the use of a larger number of objects and hiding places, as well as progressively finer tactual discriminations for their identification.

To reduce Peter's echolalic responses to comments, the experimenter modelled appropriate responses to taperecorded comments relevant to the current play situation. Peter initially imitated the experimenter's responses, which faded as Peter began to respond spontaneously to the taperecorded comments. The experimenter then facilitated an extension of Peter's appropriate comment responses to other conversational situations during a play. A detailed outline of the treatment program is found in Evans (1985).

Results

Peter's responses to the adjacency pairs included in the baseline sets were classified by the first author according to the scheme described previously. A review of

the subclassifications for responses ($N = 324$) from all baseline sessions (three pre-treatment; three during treatment; three post-treatment) yielded 97% exact intrajudge agreement. One-third of the responses ($n = 108$) were also independently coded by the second author. Interjudge agreement on sub-classifications was 92%. Disagreements were resolved prior to data analysis.

The total number of appropriate responses to all adjacency pairs increased from 42% in the three initial baselines to 66% in the three final baselines (Figure 1). Appropriate responses to each of the six adjacency pairs also increased (Table 1). Figure 2 shows that appropriate responses to the trained adjacency pairs (*Where Question-Answer, Comment-Acknowledgement*) improved by a larger amount than appropriate responses to untrained pairs.

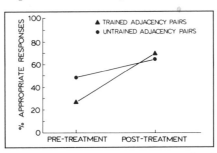

Figure 2. Appropriate responses to trained and untrained adjacency pairs.

To assess whether a significant increase in appropriate responses to the trained adjacency pairs had occurred across the intervention period, data on *Where Ques-*

tion-Answer and *Comment-Acknowledgement* adjacency pairs were combined. Each baseline elicitation sentence for the two targetted adjacency pairs ($N = 36$) was classified according to whether positive change (inappropriate to appropriate response), negative change (appropriate to inappropriate response), or no change had occurred over the intervention period. The nonparametric McNemar test for the significance of changes (Siegel, 1956) revealed that appropriate responses to trained adjacency pairs increased significantly ($X^2(1, N = 36) = 10.32, p < .001$) over the treatment period.

Unexpectedly, appropriate responses to non-trained adjacency pairs also increased—$X^2(1, N = 72) = 4.35, p < .04$. Inspection of the data suggested that improved responses to the pair *Offer-Acceptance/Rejection* were primarily responsible for the significant improvement in responses to untrained adjacency pairs. A comparison of untrained adjacency pair types omitting "offers" revealed no significant difference between pre-treatment and post-treatment accuracy measures—$X^2(1, N = 54) = 2.08, p > .05$.

Other Measures

Measures of manual searching and mitigated echolalia (Table 1) provided additional confirmation of the success of the intervention program. Peter's use of manual searching increased from 35 instances during pre-treatment baselines to 68 occurrences in the post-treatment baseline sessions. Although the overall percentage of echolalia in Peter's spontaneous speech did not change over the treatment period, a higher percentage of his echolalia involved mitigated responses, rather than exact repetitions, by the end of the program. Additional changes in Peter's language skills over the treatment period also appear in Table 1.

Discussion

The language intervention program successfully improved Peter's appropriate responses to the targetted adjacency pairs. Teaching tasks were specifically geared to two alternative strategies presumably used by blind children in acquiring language skills. The success of the intervention program suggests that, while these alternative strategies may not be necessary for blind children to acquire certain language skills, they sufficiently facilitate growth in communicative competence when used in meaningful communication contexts.

Sighted children use visual searching

and observation techniques to respond to "where" questions, but blind children often rely on manual searching to achieve the same communicative end. In this study, direct training of the alternate strategy of manual searching facilitated not only Peter's ability to respond appropriately to the *Where Question-Answer* adjacency pair, but also increased his overall spontaneous use of manual searching in appropriate communicative situations.

Initially, Peter maintained appropriate turn-taking in response to comments with another alternate strategy—echolalia. Peter's echolalic responses were modified by explicitly encouraging more appropriate responses to comments. The success of this training was shown by a dramatic improvement in appropriate responses and by Peter's spontaneous and appropriate generalization of trained responses to an untrained adjacency pair (offers) for which they were appropriate.

An increase in mitigated echolalia in Peter's spontaneous speech was another positive outcome related to the intervention program. Mitigated echolalia, in which an utterance is repeated with one or more changes (often pronoun modifications), is viewed as an initial step in the conversion of unanalyzed echolalic responses to appropriate, grammatically productive use of language (Prizant, 1982, 1983; Schuler, 1979).

A positive transfer from the intervention program did not occur for untrained adjacency pairs, with the exception of *Offer-Acknowledgement/Rejection* (see above), suggesting that the changes in responses to trained pairs could be attributed specifically to the nature of the intervention program rather than to general influences such as increased familiarity with the experimenter or increased adult attention.

Ideally, future research will establish the applicability of the present language intervention program for other blind, multiply handicapped preschoolers. In the interim, this report adds to a small, but growing, literature documenting intervention programs that effectively enhance blind children's appropriate use of language in context (Rogow, 1981, 1983).

References

Andersen, E.S., Dunlea, A., & Kekelis, L.S. (1984). Blind children's language: Resolving some differences. *Journal of Child Language, 11*, 645–664.

Anderson, G.S., & Smith, A.M. (1979). *Receptive expressive language assessment for the visually impaired*. Ingham, MI: Ingham Intermediate School District.

Bloom, L., & Lahey, M. (1978). *Language development and language disorders*. New York: John Wiley and Sons.

Brown, R. (1973). *A first language: The early stages*. Cambridge, MA: Harvard University Press.

Clark, E.V., & Sengul, C.J. (1978). Strategies in the acquisition of deixis. *Journal of Child Language, 5*, 457–475.

Clark, H.H., & Clark, E.V. (1977). *Psychology and language; An introduction to psycholinguistics*. New York: Harcourt, Brace, Jovanovich.

Cromer, R.F. (1973). Conservation by the congenitally blind. *British Journal of Psychology, 64*, 241–250.

Cromer, R.F. (1983). The implication of research findings on blind children for semantic theories and for intervention programmes. In A.E. Mills (ed.), *Language acquisition in the blind child: Normal and deficient*. San Diego: College Hill Press.

Elstner, W. (1983). Abnormalities in the verbal communication of visually impaired children. In A.E. Mills (ed.), *Language acquisition in the blind child: Normal and deficient*. San Diego: College Hill Press.

Evans, C.J. (1985). *Training pragmatic skills through alternate strategies with a blind multi-handicapped child*. Unpublished manuscript, Department of Communicative Disorders, University of Western Ontario, London, Ontario, Canada.

Fay, W.H. (1973). On the echolalia of the blind and of the autistic child. *Journal of Speech and Hearing Disorders, 38*, 478–489.

Fey, M.E. (1986). *Language intervention with young children*. San Diego: College Hill Press.

Fraiberg, S. (1977). *Insights from the blind: Development studies of blind children*. New York: Basic Books.

Ford, S. (1984). *Functions of echolalia in a blind child*. Unpublished manuscript, University of Western Ontario, London, Ontario, Canada.

Garman, M. (1983). The investigation of vision in language development. In A.E. Mills (ed.), *Language acquisition in the blind child: Normal and deficient*. San Diego: College Hill Press.

Kitzinger, M. (1984). The role of repeated and echoed utterances in communication with a blind child. *British Journal of Disorders of Communication, 19*, 135–146.

Landau, B. (1983). Blind children's language is not "meaningless." In A.E. Mills (ed.), *Language acquisition in the blind child: Normal and deficient*. San Diego: College Hill Press.

McGurk, H. (1983). Effectance motivation and the development of communicative competence in blind and sighted children. In A.E. Mills (ed.), *Language acquisition in the blind child: Normal and deficient*. San Diego: College Hill Press.

Miller, J.F. (1981). *Assessing language production in children*. Baltimore: University Park Press.

Mulford, R. (1983). Referential development in blind children. In A.E. Mills (ed.), *Language acquisition in the blind child: Normal and deficient*. San Diego: College Hill Press.

Nelson, K. (1978). Semantic development and the development of semantic memory. In K.E. Nelson (ed.), *Children's language, Volume 1*. New York: Gardner Press.

Nieuwesteeg, Y. (October, 1981). *Pragmatics in blind and sighted children*. Paper presented at the Ontario Speech and Hearing Association Convention, London, Ontario, Canada.

Piaget, J., & Inhelder, B. (1969). *The psychology of the child*. London: Routledge and Kegan-Paul.

Prizant, B.M. (1982). Speech-language pathologists and autistic children: What is our role? Part II. *American Speech and Hearing Association, 25*, 531–537.

Prizant, B.M. (1983). Language acquisition and communicative behavior in autism: Toward an understanding of the "whole" of it. *Journal of Speech and Hearing Disorders, 48*, 296–307.

Prizant, B.M., & Duchan, J.F. (1981). The functions of immediate echolalia in autistic children. *Journal of Speech and Hearing Disorders, 46*, 241–249.

Rogow, S.M. (1981). Developing play skills and communicative competence in multihandicapped young people. *Journal of Visual Impairment & Blindness, 75*, 197–202.

Rogow, S.M. (1983). Social routines and language play: Developing communication responses in developmentally delayed blind children. *Journal of Visual Impairment & Blindness, 77*, 1–4.

Schuler, A.L. (1979). Echolalia: Issues and clinical applications. *Journal of Speech and Hearing Disorders, 44*, 411–434.

Siegel, S. (1956). *Nonparametric statistics for the behavioral sciences*. New York: McGraw-Hill.

Urwin, C. (1984a). Language for absent things: Learning from visually handicapped children. *Topics in Language Disorders, 4*(4), 24–37.

Urwin, C. (1984b). Communication in infancy and the emergence of language in blind children. In R.L. Schiefelbusch & J. Pickar (eds.), *The acquisition of communicative competence*. Baltimore: University Park Press.

Wills, D. (1979). Early speech development in blind children. *Psychoanalytic Study of the Child, 34*, 85–120.

Wood, B.S. (1981). *Children and communication: Verbal and nonverbal language development* (2nd ed.). Englewood Cliffs, NJ: Prentice-Hall.

Charlotte Evans, M.Cl.Sc./CCC-SP, Manitoba School for the Deaf, 500 Shaftesbury Blvd., Winnipeg MB, R3P 0M1 Canada; Carla Johnson, M.S., 1425 Wonderland Road N., London ON, N6G 2C2, Canada.

Developing Play Skills and Communicative Competence in Multiply Handicapped Young People

S.M. Rogow

Abstract: Role play with toys was modeled to develop communicative language function in 14 multiply handicapped individuals ranging in age from 8 to 26 whose speech was characterized by echolalic and stereotypic responses. Even subjects who spoke in complete sentences asked few questions and did not use narrative speech to any significant degree. As they learned to role play, however, their communicative functioning improved and they shared referents (play themes and toy props) and cooperative social routines (role play). Play themes that were of personal interest elicited the greatest participation. Nonverbal subjects did not develop symbolic play, but they did establish communicative responses as they began to anticipate and express their preferences. No changes were noted in the verbal subjects' syntax or vocabulary. Verbal expression increased and narrative and question forms appeared. Language behavior became more communicative and meaningful as social interaction increased.

The genesis of language itself, in which the function of communication had the definite role of an essential function, presumes from the outset the existence of partners, between whom an exchange of information has taken place (Slama-Cazacu, 1977)

Communicative competence can be defined as the ability to participate in conversational dialogue, anticipate and respond to the listener's need for information, formulate and convey that information, and enjoy the reciprocity of social exchange.

Communication is the ability to transfer meaning to another person. It is a transaction—a "shared" behavior—and requires that two or more persons act as partners in an exchange of dialogue relation. Its function can be realized through any expression to another person, real or imaginary. As Slama-Cazacu (1977) pointed out, the dialogue relation begins with the simplest form of address and progresses to complex conversation, which is characterized by the presence of partners, direction toward the partner, alternate exchange, transfer of

This article is based on a research project funded by the Education Research Institute of the British Columbia Grants Program.

information, and the linguistic form in which it appears.

Multiply handicapped blind children who have not established a dialogue relation are unable to share their feelings, thoughts, needs, or desires with other people, and their language is unrelated to the immediate context. At times, they may repeat television commercials or meaningless jargon, mimic adult speech without reference to meaning, or use abusive language which they do not understand but which elicits immediate reactions from adults and/or other children. At other times, they may perseverate: e.g., ask the same question over and over again. They may use infantile pronunciation or immature expressions and incomplete sentences.

In other words, the language of multiply handicapped blind children reflects all their problems: lack of experience, disordered perceptions, inability to organize experience, hostility, anxiety, compulsiveness, and immaturity (Frampton, Kerney, & Schattner, 1969). Even when they want to communicate, they seem unable to use the language they do possess. Teachers who work with them are confronted with the problem of directing their language skills toward communicating with other people.

The communicative functions of language establish joint or common referents and referential relationships and establish joint or cooperative social routines (McLean & Snyder-McLean, 1978). The project described in this article explored the efficacy of symbolic or make-believe play as a medium for developing the communicative functions of language. In make-believe play, the referents (play objects) and cooperative social routines are clearly defined.

The continuity of conversation between two or more partners depends on the partners' attention and response to one another's requests for information, action, or confirmation. These requests, the basic components of conversation, have been termed *contingent queries* (Garvey, 1975), which depend on the situational context and are important building blocks of conversational interaction. According to Garvey, conversational partners use two kinds of contingent queries to direct and regulate the conversation: solicited and unsolicited queries. Solicited queries secure the partner's attention and encourage his or her participation. Unsolicited queries serve in cases of failures of comprehension and enable conversational partners to adjust the information to repair misunderstanding. Because contingent queries are consistent and reliable and appear so frequently in conversation, they can be used as a measure of communicative competence (Dore, 1979). By the time children are two years old, they are experienced processors of queries (Brown, 1979): i.e., they can answer and ask questions, make requests, and solicit information. The following conversation between a 26-month-old boy and his mother illustrates the contingent query (Brown, 1979): Adam (pointing to the tape recorder): "Radio." Mother: "No, tape recorder." Adam: "Tape corder?" Mother: "Yes."

The seven-month study described in this article began in April 1979 and was completed in March 1980. Play offers the blind multiply handicapped child an opportunity to experience the sharing that is involved in communication. To pretend, children must become actors. They must have a plan of action or a story line and have objects or settings that can be changed or invented as needed (Garvey, 1977). Furthermore, make-believe play enables teachers to share experiences with children, respond to their interests, and create a dialogue relation. Because conversational interaction is intrinsic to make-believe play, this type of play is an ideal medium for developing the communicative functions of language among multiply handicapped blind children. For older subjects, the play situations can be modified or adapted to meet their interests and avoid the child-like connotations of make-believe play.

The current study

The purpose of the current study was to develop or increase the conversational interactions of multiply handicapped subjects. Dialogue and conversational interaction can be actively taught to children who do not demonstrate spontaneous, self-initiated play or express interest in social interaction. Creating situations that involve shared social routines can bring the language abilities of noncommunicating children under social control and develop conversational skills. To achieve this goal, the study was divided into two parts. In the first part, the responses of subjects to play situations created by teachers were analyzed; the second part involved a more formal investigation of the changes that occurred in the subjects' linguistic behavior. Samples of the language used by the subjects were obtained at the beginning of the study and at four-week intervals throughout the seven months.

As shown in Table 1, subjects—eight, ages 8 to 12; five teenagers; and one 26-year-old—participated in the study (all names are fictitious). Six subjects were totally blind, three were partially blind, and five were sighted. Sighted children were included in the study because their language difficulties resembled those of the visually impaired subjects. All subjects had additional disabilities such as mental retardation, cerebral palsy, or emotional disturbance. Ten youngsters were referred by teachers or school administrators; three were referred by nurses on wards for severely handicapped individuals at a large provincial institution for the mentally retarded. One severely disabled sighted child was included in the study at his mother's request.

At the beginning of the study, each subject's level of language development was categorized according to the following stages (Crystal, Fletcher, & Garman, 1976):

No verbal language. Speech is not used to indicate needs or wants.

Stage I. One-element utterances: e.g., "Mommy," "shoe."

Stage II. Two-element phrases: e.g., "shoe there," "Daddy come."

Stage III. Three-element phrases; beginning use of plurals, pronouns, and possessives: e.g., "Daddy's shoes," "my ball."

Stage IV. Simple sentence constructions; true grammar represented by word order, verb tenses, articles, and auxiliaries; and pronouns, adjectives, and major parts of speech present.

Stage V. Compound and complex sentence constructions; connecting

Table 1. Characteristics of Subjects (N=14).

Name	Age	Sex	Visual status	Cause of visual impairment	Additional handicaps[a]	Stage of language development	Type of educational program
Alice	14	F	Totally blind	RLF	Mild emotional disturbance	VI	Special class
Betty	12	F	Partially sighted	Aneridia	Mild emotional disturbance; mild mental retardation; mild cultural deprivation	V	Special class
Charles	14	M	Partially sighted	Cataracts	Moderate emotional disturbance; mild mental retardation	VI	Special class
Donald	9	M	Totally blind	RLF	Cerebral palsy; spastic quadraplegia; epilepsy; moderate mental retardation	IV	Special school (MR)
Ed	26	M	Totally blind	RLF	Moderate emotional disturbance; epilepsy; moderate mental retardation	II	None
Frances	17	F	Totally blind	Unknown	Mild emotional disturbance; spastic quadraplegia; moderate mental retardation	II	None
Gail	17	F	Partially sighted	Cataracts	Mild emotional disturbance; moderate mental retardation; mild cultural deprivation	IV	Special school (MR)
Henry	12	M	Sighted		Mild emotional disturbance; moderate mental retardation	III	Special school (MR)
Irene	14	F	Sighted		Moderate mental retardation	III	Special school (MR)
Jane	8	F	Totally blind	Unknown	Trigeminal nerve damage; severe mental retardation	No speech	None
Kenneth	8	M	Totally blind	Trauma	Spastic quadraplegia; severe mental retardation	No speech	Special school (MR)
Lyle	8	M	Sighted		Spastic quadraplegia; severe mental retardation	No speech	None
Mike	11	M	Sighted		Moderate emotional disturbance; hyperactivity; severe mental retardation	II	Special school (MR)
Nick	9	M	Sighted		Moderate emotional disturbance; hyperactivity (autistic behavior); severe mental retardation	IV	Special school (MR)

[a]Terminology used in psychological assessments of all subjects enrolled in educational programs was obtained from school records.

devices such as "and" and "but" are used.

Stage VI. Adult speech; process of acquisition is completed.

Stage VII. Discursive structure and style.

Despite differences in age and types of disabilities, all subjects exhibited limited stereotyped responses and an inability to interact meaningfully with peers, use play materials, or occupy themselves without adult direction. The verbal subjects appeared to be extremely anxious about interacting with peers: They demonstrated little narrative or conversational speech, asked almost no questions, and their verbal expressions were stereotyped or were related more to their own anxieties and concerns than to events occurring around them. They showed little curiosity or imagination in their verbal expressions and sought reassurance rather than information.

Baseline information on each subject's play behavior was gathered from two sources: classroom teachers and ward staff. Each subject was then involved in an informal play session.

During the initial sessions, subjects were allowed to choose from a variety of toys such as baby dolls, Barbie dolls, stuffed animals, hand and string puppets, toy furniture, and appliances—all of which clearly called for imaginative themes. The teachers encouraged them to explore the toys by making comments such as, "Here's a doll" or "What can you do with this toy?" but did not show them how to play with the toys. Although these sessions may not have reflected the childrens' skills accurately because of the newness of the situation and lack of play experiences, all the blind and visually impaired subjects and one sighted subject seemed to be at a loss as to what to do with the play materials. They either rejected the toys or handled them only briefly. One sighted subject began to play with the toys, but his play was solitary and did not involve language.

Those toys that represented familiar objects were chosen most frequently. Nonverbal subjects were most occupied with toys that had novel elements and appealed to the senses of touch and hearing. Older subjects selected Barbie dolls and well-made string or hand puppets.

Play sessions

In the play segment of the project, each subject played alone with a teacher-model at least one hour each week (total play time, 28 hours). The teacher-models were two graduate students (one, a head teacher at a school for trainable mentally retarded children) and nine student teachers enrolled in a teacher education program for the visually impaired at the University of British Columbia. The play sessions conducted for the seven youngsters enrolled at the school for the mentally retarded were conducted twice a week for 15 to 45 minutes. At all other settings, the play sessions took place once a week for at least one hour.

The teachers were alone with the subjects during the play sessions. Each teacher kept detailed records of each play session. In addition, a play progress chart was kept on each subject, four sessions were tape recorded, and each subject was videotaped.

Language samples were taken at four-week intervals throughout the project. The initial language samples indicated few question forms or requests for information, action, or confirmation (contingent queries). (More detailed information about the subjects' language development appears in the discussion about Part II.)

Participation in play

Extent of participation is a measure of the involvement of the child in play. To record changes in participatory behavior, four levels of participation were used:
• passive participation: The subject was a spectator and indicated interest by laughing, smiling, or commenting.
• active imitation. The subject began to imitate the action of play through a motor action, an action with a toy prop, or verbal imitation of the adult.
• active participation in thematic play: The subject added to the theme set by the teacher through ideas, motor behavior, verbal expression, or role.
• subject-initiated theme: The subject developed his own play theme and initiated the play.

All subjects were participating in the play sessions when the project ended. Most began with passive participation. The blind subjects initially needed a great deal of encouragement and experience in using the toys before they could actively participate or use the toy props in an imaginative way. All verbal subjects moved quickly from passive participation to active participation in a play theme. Most subjects did not plan their own play themes. Unless the teachers developed a theme, the children repeated the themes of the previous session. The teachers had

to elaborate on or change a theme to challenge the children to incorporate new or novel material. This was as true of those children with a high level of linguistic skills as those with limited skills. Children with well-developed skills did not generate their own ideas without a good deal of prompting and elaborating by teachers. Nevertheless, most eventually began to contribute ideas, role characterizations, feelings, and solutions to problems posed by the teachers.

The actual toy props became less and less important as the subjects became more willing and more expert at "pretending" situations. For example, when Ed's puppet spilled "pretend" ketchup all over its tie and the teacher asked him to help clean it up, Ed wiped the stain from the puppet's "pretend" tie. When Betty's teacher said that the dolls were fighting over some crayons, Betty solved the problem by adding more "pretend" crayons "so each doll will have her own." Irene chased away a cow that was nibbling on her sandwich. When Alice realized that she could control the lives of her dolls, she began to express genuine feelings: She comforted her puppet by saying, "If you need help, you can ask for it. You have to know when you need help." Charles, who was anxious about a pending airplane trip, acted out the sequence of taking a trip: he called a taxi to take him to the airport, boarded an airplane, ate his dinner, landed, and met his aunt at the airport.

Symbolic behavior

Before symbolic behavior could be established, the subjects had to explore repeatedly to become familiar with the toys and how they could be used. The fact that children who showed greatest interest in interacting socially with their teachers made the most rapid progress in developing exploratory play skills suggests that objects assume importance in relation to the personal satisfaction with which they are associated.

All subjects had to become familiar with the toys before they could use them symbolically. Few differences were observed between blind and sighted subjects in the way they used the toys once they were familiar with them. The sighted subjects quickly recognized familiar characters such as Donald Duck and Mickey Mouse, but their attention was fleeting and they rarely used the toys appropriately until their exploratory skills were well established. Attention to the toy was facilitated by playing with it. Once the subjects had learned how to act upon a toy, they began to use it more actively. Playing with toys involves more than simple action on an object. A toy is embellished with a purpose. Random handling or whirling and other forms of stereotypic behavior with the toys diminished as actions became purposeful.

At first, the three nonverbal subjects—two totally blind and one sighted child—refused to participate at all. They either threw the toys on the floor or clenched their fists and refused to touch them. As they became familiar with the routine of the sessions and began to anticipate interacting with their teachers, they became interested in the toys.

This observation suggests once again that social interaction is important in fostering interest in objects. The teachers taught the children how to explore and manipulate the toy props by guiding their hands with their own. The nonverbal children tended to treat the toys as objects to be handled for their sensory attributes rather than as tools or as representative of real objects. They handled dolls, trucks, and dishes the same way. The nonverbal children became interested in the actions they discovered they could perform.

Although none of these children developed symbolic behavior, they did exhibit anticipation and expressed their preferences. In other words, they learned to imitate the teachers' motor behavior with toy props.

The symbolic behavior of play, "pretending," can take many forms. Pretending is a cognitive activity, and before children can portray or represent an action or object, they must possess an image or notion of it. There was variation among the subjects in the use of symbolic behavior. The pretending of some children was limited to representing physical actions such as eating, running, dancing, jumping, and the like. All the verbal subjects demonstrated some progress in the ways they combined ideas and objects. Interest in the toy props and familiarity with the play themes suggested by the teachers appeared to be important elements in encouraging the children to participate actively in play. The teachers made many false starts while trying to identify the interests of individual children. Themes that were important and familiar to the children evoked the greatest intensity and absorption. The child's own interests were critical factors in the depth and intensity of play. These interests ranged from motor activities, such as driving a car, to emotionally charg-

ed situations such as going to the doctor or moving to a new school.

Changes were noted in the use of the toy props. As the play sessions developed, fewer toys were needed to keep the play themes going. More objects and situations could be imagined, but dolls that were characters in a play had to be present at all times.

Materials such as tea sets, grocery items, and dolls and puppets evoked more imaginary uses than did stuffed animals, trucks, and baby strollers. The nonverbal children responded most to toys that provided pleasurable sounds and textures. Although sighted children were initially able to recognize objects more easily than were visually impaired children, once object recognition was accomplished, the differences diminished. Realism and familiarity of toy props were important to all subjects.

With the exception of subjects whose language was most advanced, both visually impaired and sighted subjects enjoyed the representation of motor action in play. This was especially noticeable in blind subjects who had other physical disabilities. Donald, who had other severe physical handicaps in addition to blindness, enjoyed rocking his body while pretending to drive a car. Frances rocked her own body while rocking her "baby" to sleep.

Linguistically advanced subjects were most involved in the dialogue involved in play and paid more attention to role characterization, problem-solving, and the aggression of feelings.

Role play
According to Garvey (1977), children assume three kinds of roles during play: 1) functional roles defined by the action theme of the play: e.g., if there is a car, there must be a driver; 2) speaking for a doll or stuffed toy animal; and 3) character roles defined by occupation: e.g., doctor, mommy, daddy, baby—roles that tend to be associated with appropriate actions and differ from functional roles in that they can be adopted without taking part in any action.

All subjects engaged in the three types of role play. Functional roles predominated among subjects with Stage III language development or less. Those with the most advanced language development were most able to assume character roles defined by dialogue rather than motor activity. All verbal subjects, however, responded to the character roles assumed

by the teachers: i.e., they were not disturbed or confused when teachers pretended to be a doll or a toy animal or slipped in and out of a play role. They also understood that when the teachers changed their normal tone of voice and expression, they were characterizing a play role. Some children began to imitate the teachers' expressions and changed their normal way of talking.

Even when the children did assume a character role, they had difficulty playing a role that was not themselves. Initially, dialogue took the form of conversational responses to the role the teachers played.

As the play sessions progressed, the children's role characterizations became more vivid and expressive. Gail interacted with three Barbie dolls as though they were able to reply to her and changed her tone of voice while pretending that she was their mother or teacher. She addressed each doll by name and directed her attention to the doll when it "spoke."
Gail: Listen to me. I am talking to you. Eat it, the food on the plate. Drink the cup through the mouth.

Are you having a nice time? Yeah! By listening, you can talk. (Turning to teacher) My friends listen to me and they talk to me.

Irene portrayed herself while pretending to have a picnic in the park. Despite her limited vocabulary and fluency, she could portray a role vividly:
Teacher: Are you dressed warmly enough?
Irene: No, cold.
Teacher: Here is your sweater. Are you warm enough now?
Irene: No, coat?
Teacher: O.K. but you get it.
Irene: Oh, heavy.
Teacher: Is it too heavy?
Irene: Too heavy.

There was a definite shift away from pure description of actions or toy props to interpreting and acting out real life roles. Teachers played a critical and sensitive role in facilitating dialogue. If they were too active, a child was placed in the role of the audience; if they were not active enough, they failed to define and elicit active participation. Teachers also found that it was important to shift their roles to avoid stereotypic or routine responses.

Changes in linguistic behavior
As mentioned earlier, 11 subjects were verbal when the study began: two used adult speech; one spoke in compound and complex sentences; three, in simple sentences; and five, in two- or three-word phrases.

Regardless of their level of syntactic development, however, they asked few questions and seldom made contingent queries or personal comments or used narrative or descriptive speech.

Method

To assess the nature of the changes that occurred in the subjects' linguistic behavior, all play sessions were recorded and transcribed into scripts. The teacher-subject conversational interactions of four play sessions for each subject were transcribed at two-month intervals. The 44 transcriptions were then analyzed using the following measures of conversational interaction: 1) frequency of requests for action or confirmation (contingent queries), 2) frequency of replies to teachers' queries, 3) frequency of nonresponses to teachers' queries, and 4) frequency of conversational acts (dyadic interchanges) in a single session.

Table 2. Number of queries made by verbal subjects during play sessions (at two-month intervals).

Subject	Month 1	Month 3	Month 5	Month 7
Alice	2	3	6	8
Betty	2	3	4	3
Charles	1	2	2	2
Donald	2	4	2	7
Ed	0	0	0	0
Frances	0	0	0	0
Gail	4	8	12	11
Henry	0	0	0	3
Irene	0	0	4	4
Mean	1.3	2.2	3.3	4.5

Table 3. Number of replies to teachers' queries over seven months.

Subject	Month 1	Month 3	Month 5	Month 7
Alice	6	6	12	14
Betty	4	4	9	7
Charles	9	6	11	7
Donald	4	4	6	8
Ed	2	0	9	7
Frances	1	0	4	8
Gail	5	8	16	9
Henry	6	10	12	8
Irene	7	8	12	14
Mean	4.9	5.1	10.1	9.1

As illustrated in Table 2, the average number of queries made by verbal subjects increased from 1.3 to 4.5 per session over the seven-month period. Table 3 shows that a substantial mean increase also occurred in the subjects' replies to queries

from teachers (from 4.9 to 9.1). Note in Table 4 that there was a corresponding decline in the number of nonresponses to teachers' queries over the seven months (1.8 to 0.6). The increase in nonresponses during the third month may reflect the teachers' lack of familiarity with the subjects and their interests and an improvement in the quality of the teachers' queries as the teachers became more familiar with the subjects' interests.

Table 4. Nonresponses to teacher questions over seven months.

Subject	Month 1	Month 3	Month 5	Month 7
Alice	0	0	0	0
Betty	3	6	2	0
Charles	2	1	1	1
Donald	4	7	0	0
Ed	0	0	3	0
Frances	3	4	3	3
Gail	2	1	1	0
Henry	2	2	3	0
Irene	0	1	0	1
Totals	16	22	13	5
Mean	1.8	2.4	1.4	0.6

Table 5. Increase in dyadic interchanges between subjects and teachers over seven months.

Subject	Month 1	Month 3	Month 5	Month 7
Alice	11	16	24	32
Betty	8	8	13	18
Charles	3	4	8	12
Donald	2	4	7	14
Ed	4	5	8	9
Frances	4	3	8	9
Gail	8	11	14	18
Henry	8	10	38	41
Irene	14	19	24	27
Mean	6.9	8.9	16.0	20.0

Table 5 indicates the number of dyadic interchanges that took place in each of the four taped play sessions. Note that the average number of dyadic interchanges had increased from approximately 7 to 20 by the end of the project. Also note that all subjects improved markedly in this area over the seven months: The number of interchanges increased two- to six-fold.

Discussion

Dramatic play provides a motivating structure for eliciting communicative behavior. The opportunities for social interaction provided during the play sessions directed the subjects' language into social channels. Dialogue developed in play situations in

which the subjects were treated as equal partners whose ideas were encouraged and who functioned co-actively.

Both play and language are social behavior. The children who most enjoyed social interactions with the teachers became the most effective and imaginative players. Level of syntactic development was not a determinant in either the richness of subjects' play dialogue or the intensity of their participation.

The results of this study suggest that symbolic play has an important function in the development of communicative competence. Conversation, social interaction, imagination, social awareness, and a sense of shared pleasure can be derived from play. The conceptual (symbolic) and communicative (dialogue) functions of language are enriched and expanded in play. The simultaneous development of language and imagination is seen in the play of young children. Special education for severely disabled children can profitably take the form of increasing and developing play skills in blind children with additional handicaps, who do not demonstrate spontaneous play.

References

Brown, R. (1976). *A first language: The early stages.* Harmondsworth, England: Penguin Books.

Crystal, D., Fletcher, P., & Garman, M. (1976). *The grammatical analysis of language disability.* London, England: Edward Arnold.

Dore, J. (1979). Conversational acts and the acquisition of language. In E. Ochs and B.B. Schieffelin (eds.), *Developmental pragmatics.* New York: Academic Press.

Frampton, M.E., Kerney, E., & Schattner, R. (1969). *Forgotten children: A program for the multihandicapped.* Boston: Porter-Sargent.

Garvey, C. (1975). Requests and responses in children's speech. *Journal of Child Language, 2,* 41-64.

Garvey, C. (1977). *Play.* Cambridge, MA: Harvard University Press.

McLean, J.E. & Snyder-McLean, L.K. (1978). *A transactional approach to early language training.* New York: Charles E. Merrill.

Piaget, J. (1962). *Play, dreams and imitation in childhood.* New York: W.W. Norton.

Slama-Cazacu, T. (1977). *Dialogue in children.* The Hague, The Netherlands: Mouton Publishers.

Sally M. Rogow, Ed.D., associate professor and coordinator, Diploma Program in the Education of the Visually Impaired, University of British Columbia, Vancouver, British Columbia, Canada.

ENVIRONMENTS

Attention to the most meaningful features of the environment is essential for the individual whose senses limit information. These articles focus on aspects of perceiving the environment which are functional for the visually impaired person with multiple handicaps, and they detail processes for learning to use the senses effectively.

Teaching Visual Attention in Functional Contexts: Acquisition and Generalization of Complex Visual Motor Skills

L. Goetz; K. Gee

Abstract: A three-year-old girl with multiple severe disabilities including aphakia was taught to visually attend to stimulus items in a training program that emphasized functional, age-appropriate visual motor tasks that required the use of vision for successful task completion. Within these task contexts, use of a repeated prompting procedure was successful in establishing visual attention, and generalization of visual attention to untrained tasks was observed. Additionally, increases in visual attention, whether trained or generalized, were associated with improved motor skill accuracy in the absence of any direct motor skill training on several tasks. Results are discussed in terms of classroom implications for vision "stimulation" programs and in terms of visual attention as a critical skill that may show multiple treatment effects.

Several reports have documented changes in visual behaviors of multiply handicapped students as a function of contingent consequences (Maier & Hogg, 1974; Utley, Duncan, Strain, & Scanlon, 1984). While these reports are promising, numerous questions are also raised by the existing literature. Procedurally, the use of artifical positive reinforcement (e.g., reinforcing looking at an instructional stimulus with the delivery of an edible reinforcer) fails to teach the student the natural contingencies and consequences of visual attention. Presumably, generalization and long-term maintenance of visual attention learned through instruction will ultimately depend upon the natural, not the artificial, consequences of vision use.

A second critical issue is the failure of the available literature to analyze the relationship between functional visual attention and skill performance. Does teaching a student to use his vision efficiently affect actual task performance? The crucial role of visually attending to instructional

stimuli seems obvious, yet those investigators who have established visual behaviors in their subjects (Craig & Holland, 1970) have failed to document whether or not increased visual attention actually affected performance on the task(s) to which the student was attending.

Thus, the purposes of the current pilot study were twofold: 1) to evaluate the hypothesis that a contingent, "functional context" training program that utilized natural consequences rather than artificial reinforcers could be effective in establishing generalized visual attention to training stimuli; and 2) to provide an analysis of the relationship between learned visual attention skills and performance of other skills in the training context.

Method

Subject and setting

Lisa was a three-year-old, nonambulatory girl with severe retardation who was attending her first preschool intervention program. Lisa's visual status included congenital cataracts and glaucoma. Her cataracts had been surgically removed and she wore glasses to correct her resulting aphakia. Accurate visual acuity measures had been sought, but the outcome was reported as "unable to evaluate." Lisa clearly functioned as if she had residual vision; she would visually search for and

find food items that fell from her plate during lunch. She also crawled and/or scooted about the room without running into major obstacles.

The setting in which the study took place was a public school model classroom serving nine severely handicapped and deaf/blind students. All instructional procedures were carried out at a small table in the classroom as part of regularly scheduled classroom activities.

Task selection and dependent measures

Six tasks were selected as meeting three criteria for "functional context" training: 1) All tasks inherently required visual attention to be completed successfully; 2) all tasks were functional (they increased independence in present and future environments); and 3) all tasks were age-appropriate for the student (Brown et al., 1980).

For each task, a "critical moment" was determined. The critical moment was defined as the time during task performance when continuous eye contact or fixation on the task materials was necessary to correctly complete the task; i.e., to correctly hang a cup on a hook, one need not look continuously at the cup while picking it up and directing it toward the hook; however, one must look at both stimulus items while actually positioning and slipping the handle over the hook. The six tasks and their critical visual moments are presented in Table 1.

Two dependent measures were recorded: visual attention to the task and accuracy of task performance. Each trial had a maximum 30-minute duration that began with the initial instructional cue. During a trial, visual attention was defined as continuous eye contact with the materials *during the critical moment* of the task. If the student looked at the materials during the critical moment, regardless of actual task performance, a plus was scored. If the student looked at the materials initially, but stopped looking at the critical moment, visual attention was scored as a minus.

Accuracy of task performance was defined as successful completion of the motor task, and was scored independently of visual attention.

Design and procedures

A multiple-baseline, multiple-probe (Farb & Throne, 1978; Horner & Baer, 1978) design across six tasks within subjects was used.

Baseline

The task materials were presented, and the instructor requested, "Look and do x." No instruction occurred and social reinforce-

This research was supported in part by USOE contract #G300-78-0338, and in part by USOE Grant #G008300032. Special thanks are extended to Tom Haring for his comments on prior versions of this manuscript. Portions of this paper were presented at the Tenth Annual Conference of The Association for Persons with Severe Handicaps, Chicago, 1984.

Table 1. Functional visual motor tasks and critical visual moments.

Task	Critical Moment
1. insert puzzle piece	—from time of positioning over hole to completing insertion
2. stack rings over pole	—from time ring touches pole (or is centrally positioned) to complete stacking
3. put lid on pot	—from time lid touches rim of pot (or is centrally positioned) to completing insertion
4. stack glasses	—from time glass touches rim of other glass (or is centrally positioned) to completing insertion
5. insert coin in piggy bank	—from time coin is within 1″ of slot to completion of insertion
6. hang cup on hook	—while slipping handle over hook

the first ten sessions of baseline on all tasks, performance seldom rose above 10 percent. For the first two skills (complete puzzle and stack ring), skill training alone also failed to affect looking behavior, although a slight upward trend occurred for skill 1. However, the success of the visual attention training procedure in establishing visual attending is reflected in the relatively abrupt rise in looking behavior each time the procedure was introduced for these two tasks.

ment was delivered noncontingently. A trial lasted 30 minutes.

Skill training

The instructor delivered the same cue as in baseline. If the student correctly performed the task (regardless of visual attention), she was socially reinforced and allowed to play briefly with a favored toy. If the response was incorrect, it was scored as such, and she was fully assisted to perform the motor task. However, no procedures were used to establish visual attention.

Visual attention training

During this phase, a repeated prompting procedure (Koegel & Egel, 1978; Utley, 1979) was used to establish visual attention. This procedure involved repeating the verbal cue and adding a necessary prompt (loudly tapping with an index finger the critical location on the item where Lisa was required to look) as many times as needed until visual attention was established. If Lisa attempted to complete the tasks without visual attention, her task response was interrupted and she was not allowed to continue until visual attention was established. Once established, if Lisa stopped visually attending, visual attention was again re-established as often as needed until the 30 minutes of the trial ran out. Thus, the opportunity to perform the motor task was contingent upon first visually attending to it. No other reinforcement procedures were used.

Reliability

Twenty-six interobserver reliability checks were taken by an independent observer. The range was .70-1.00, with a mean of .97 and a median of 1.0.

Results

Results are presented in figure 1.

Visual attention training

The initial baseline data for visual attention indicate that Lisa failed to look while attempting to do any of the tasks. During

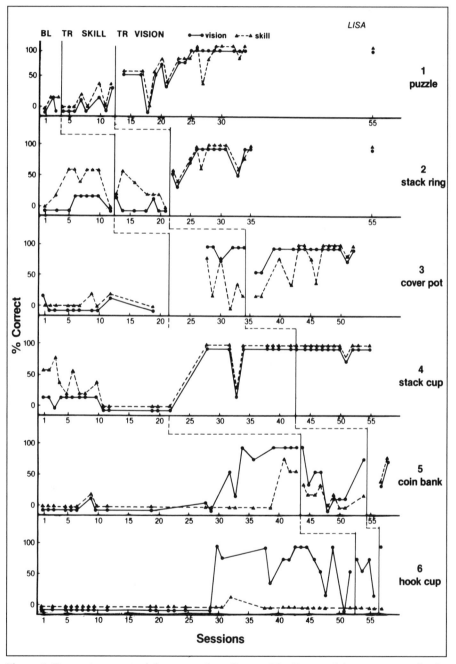

Figure 1. Percent correct trials per session. ●━━━━━● indicates vision responses (looking during the "critical moment" of the motor task; ▲┄┄┄┄▲ represents accuracy of task performance.

These data also suggest that once visual attending was established on the first two exemplars (Session 25), generalized visual attending occurred on the remaining tasks. Both skill 3 (cover pot) and skill 4 (stack cups) show an abrupt rise in looking behavior as of session 25, and further generalization occurs gradually and successively on skills 5 (coin in bank) and 6 (cup on hook). Interestingly, this generalization effect occurred both in the presence and absence of a prior skill training alone phase (skill 3 versus skills 4-6, respectively).

Skill training

The skill acquisition data in Figure 1 indicate some variation in the accuracy of skill performance during the initial baseline phase. However, for every skill, skill training alone has no effect upon improving skill accuracy and, in fact, appears to have decreased skill performance on skill 3 and to have decreased both skill performance and visual attention on skill 5. In addition, skill training does not appear to have had significant positive effects upon visual attention.

Visual attention and skill accuracy

In contrast to the effects of skill training upon skill performance, vision training does appear to have an effect upon skill performance. The data in Figure 1 suggest co-occurrence of visual attention and accurate skill performance. For skill 3, generalized looking corresponded with an initial improvement in skill accuracy, but direct training of visual attention was needed before skill accuracy reached criterion. For skill 4, untrained looking appears to have a direct effect upon skill accuracy. Once the student looked (session 25), skill performance improved to 100 percent accuracy and both behaviors remained at high levels without any direct training. A similar trend is indicated for skill 5, although the skill training phase interrupted this trend.

Finally, the data from skill 6 suggest that while visual attention training improved skill performance, this phenomenon may be specific to skills which are not too difficult for the student to perform. For skill 6, a difficult motor task of hanging cups

on hooks, visual attention alone, generalized by day 45, did not appear sufficient to result in successful skill performance. When visual attention did not covary with improved skill performance, it appears to have undergone extinction and the student ceased to look during performance of this particular task.

Discussion

The present results, limited to a single-case investigation, are preliminary in nature and replication is clearly desirable. Nevertheless, outcomes of the current investigation suggest several implications. First, the results document that visual attention is in fact an operant behavior, and one that can be learned and maintained through application of contingent, truly functional, natural consequences. The procedures utilized in this investigation did not rely upon extrinsic artifical reinforcement for looking behaviors; the major consequence for visual attention was the opportunity to do a task, and (as a result of looking) to do it correctly.

The current findings also suggest that visual attention may be a "target skill" that has multiple treatment effects (Rincover, 1981). The finding that teaching a visual skill can result in concomitant skill acquisition of other skills without direct training of these others skills provides important empirical support to the theoretical assumption that visual attention is critical to learning (cf. Santestefano & Stayton, 1967; Barraga, 1970).

Lastly, an efficient classroom teaching procedure for teaching looking behavior has been initially identified. In order to maximize the effects of such a functional context training program, additional research is needed to further clarify both the parameters of functional skill contexts and the range of visual behaviors for which such a procedure is effective. The current data are an encouraging start.

References

Barraga, N. (1970). Teacher's guide for the development of visual learning abilities and utilization of low vision. American Printing House for the Blind.

Brown, L., Branston, M., Baumgart, D., Vincent, L., Falvey, M., & Schroeder, J. (1980). Utilizing characteristics of a variety of current and subsequent least restrictive environments as factors in development of curricular content for severely handicapped students. In L. Brown, M. Falvey, D. Baumgart, I. Pumpian, J. Schroeder, & L. Gruenwald (eds.), *Strategies for teaching chronological age-appropriate functional skills to adolescent and young adult severely handicapped students*, Vol. IX, Part 1. Madison, WI: University of Wisconsin & Madison Metropolitan School District.

Craig, H. & Holland, A. (1970). Reinforcement of visual attending in classrooms for deaf children. *Journal of Applied Behavior Analysis*, 3, 97-109.

Farb, J. & Throne, J. (1978). Improving the generalized mnemonic performance of a Down syndrome child. *Journal of Applied Behavior Analysis,* 11,, 413-420.

Horner, R.D. & Baer, D. (1978). Multiple probe technique: A variation on the multiple baseline. *Journal of Applied Behavior Analysis*, 11, 189-196.

Maier, I. & Hogg, J. (1974). The operant conditioning of sustained visual fixation in hyperactive severely retarded children. *American Journal of Mental Deficiency*, 79, 297-304.

Rincover, A. (1981). Some directions for analysis and intervention in developmental disabilities: An editorial. *Analysis and Intervention in Developmental Disabilities*, 1, 109-115.

Santostefano, S. & Stayton, S. (1967). Training the pre-school retarded child in focusing attention. A program for parents. *American Journal of Orthopyschiatry3*, 37, 732-743.

Schroeder, S. & Holland, J. (1968). The operant control of eye movements. *Journal of Applied Behavior Analysis*, 1, 161-166.

Utley, B. (1979). Annual Report: The Bay Area Severely Handicapped Deaf-Blind Project. USOE contract #300-78-0338.

Utley, B., Duncan, D., Strain, P., & Scanlon, K. (1983). Effects of contingent and noncontingent vision stimulation on visual fixation in multiply handicapped children. *Journal of the Association for Persons with Severe Handicaps*, 8, 29-42.

Lori Goetz, Ph.D., Kathleen Gee, M.A., Dept. of Special Education, San Francisco State University, 1600 Holloway Avenue, San Francisco, CA 94132.

Uses of Mechanical Vibration in the Education of Multiply Handicapped Blind Children

V. Hobbis; T. Williams

Abstract: Multiply handicapped blind children, particularly those with severe or profound mental and/or auditory handicaps, are effectively deprived of many sensations, and hence many opportunities for learning. It is therefore of particular interest when a technique is developed that appears to utilize an intact portion of their sensorium. In this paper, the uses of mechanical vibration for stimulating, rewarding and suppressing the behaviors of multiply handicapped children are discussed. A review of the published literature, together with our experience, indicate how the use of mechanical vibration has helped to develop new skills for multiply handicapped children. Suggestions for further research and refinement of the techniques are made.

Mechanical vibration as a reward technique used with handicapped people was first reported in the early 1960s. Rice and McDaniel (1960) found that "negative patients" would make simple motor responses if rewarded with films, music or vibration. Although studies with profoundly mentally handicapped people showed beneficial effects, it was not clear from these early reports whether people with sensory handicaps would be prompted to learn new skills using mechanical vibration. There are, however, reasons for suspecting that the use of vibratory stimulation of the skin might be useful, since touch has often played an important role in the education of blind persons (e.g., the Braille system), and the deaf-blind (e.g., Helen Keller's experiences). Developments in the 1970s have led to a certain degree of optimism with regard to the use of mechanical vibration in the education of multiply handicapped people, yet it has rarely formed an integral part of a teaching system, but rather has remained an adjunct (Glover & Mesibov, 1978). In this paper the value of mechanical vibration is more clearly defined and consequently, its use may be integrated more effectively into the teaching programs of the multiply handicapped child.

Vibration as a stimulus

Vibration can be used both as a stimulus indicating that something is about to happen or it may be used to stimulate the child into activity. Jones (1980) describes the use of two-minute bursts of vibration in eliciting activity in a severely quadriplegic, epileptic adolescent. Following a period allowed for the subject to settle into a comfortable chair, each burst of vibration was accompanied by an increase in eye movements, neck movements and frequency of vocalizations. In the same paper, Jones reports certain general findings regarding the use of vibration in the same way. It seems that the initial period of vibration in any one session produces the greatest effects, subsequent applications being less effective. However, if on the following day vibration is used again, there seems to be as powerful an effect as occurred on the first occasion. Different types of vibration produce different effects within the individual child. Thus, one patient may be soothed at one particular frequency or amplitude of vibration and yet be stimulated into activity by another. There are also differences between individuals in their responses to vibration. It is therefore vital to carry out a full assessment of the child's responses, using a full range of frequencies and amplitudes.

The use of vibration as a means of signaling events does not appear to have been described in the literature, but this might prove to be useful as a means of signaling the imminence of preferred activities or events. Anecdotal evidence suggests that naturally occurring vibration can be used by some of the multiply handicapped children at the Mary Sheridan Unit in this way. For instance, some children will react to someone walking towards them when they are lying on a hollow but carpeted wooden platform. The carpet deadens the sound of the footfalls but transmits the vibration.

Learning new skills

Vibration has been used as a reward in programs to teach fine-motor, gross-motor and communication skills. The essential feature of all these studies is that vibration is presented to the child immediately after a task is completed. In this respect it resembles the early studies of vibration such as those carried out by Rice and McDaniel (1960).

Jones (1980) compares the effects of sips of coffee and vibration as rewards for holding on to objects with a 13-year-old blind, mentally and physically handicapped girl. Vibration proved considerably more effective than sips of coffee, which had hitherto been considered the only effective reward for her. She learned to hold onto objects for up to 70 seconds, whereas previously she would not hold on for more than 10 seconds. Goodall et al. (1982) compared vibration and social praise with social praise alone and found that for most of the children the use of vibration enhanced the rate at which they learned to place shapes into the insets of the formboard. The authors have used vibration to teach multiply handicapped children standing and walking as well as elements of a standard sign language, with considerable success.

The use of vibration as a reward for gross-motor skills has been greatly aided by specially built equipment. In essence, this equipment automates the delivery of the reward. Thus, if the task is to walk, the equipment consists of a platform with a series of microswitches arranged so that the vibration starts only if a step forward is taken. The authors have not yet been able to assess formally whether vibration is more effective than other rewards.

Vibration as a suppressant of stereotypical behavior

As has been noted previously, Jones (1980) found that at certain frequencies and amplitudes, vibration caused multiply handicapped children to stop moving. For other children vibration seemed to act as an unpleasant stimulus, in that they would seek ways of avoiding the stimulus or of turning it off. Goodall and Corbett (1982) also showed that in certain circumstances the effect of vibration was to reduce the frequency of certain behaviors. Thus, when vibration was used as a reward for the successful completion of a task, the frequency of stereotypical behavior decreased as compared with a condition in which the reward did not include vibration.

When children with sensory impairments are engaged in repetitive or stereotyped behavior patterns, it can be very difficult to obtain their cooperation in order to teach them new skills. If sensory input can be controlled by the teacher, it should be possible to divert the child's attention more easily onto the task that is being taught.

This has been the rationale behind studies on the suppression of stereotypical behavior at the Mary Sheridan Unit. In one case, the authors demonstrated that vibration suppressed the stereotypical behaviors of a multiply handicapped 13-year-old boy. More importantly, the effect of suppressing the vibrations generalized to sessions in which no vibration was available. In another case, vibration proved somewhat less effective with a boy whose mannerisms centered on small objects. Thus when the boy had such an object, vibration had no effect on the frequency of stereotypical movements, but as soon as it was taken away, vibration suppressed the behaviors.

A few words of caution

Vibration is unlikely to be effective for all children who fail to respond to more conventional rewards. One possibility is that vibration is more appropriate for the more developmentally delayed children, and there is some evidence that this is so

(Byrne & Stevens, 1980). On the other hand, Hogg (1983) showed that vibration had little effect on the behavior of a profoundly mentally handicapped blind child. Goodall & Corbett (1982) found that those children with behavior problems were less interested in sensory stimulation such as vibration. Visually handicapped children need to be carefully assessed before vibration is used in a teaching program. In particular, if vibration is to be used to relax spastic muscles, then the advice of a qualified physioherapist should be sought, in order that no damage is caused.

The place of vibration in education

Uses of vibration have been shown in the education of the visually handicapped child with additional handicaps. However, its use in the education of such children is rare. The initial stages need not be costly exercises. Simple, battery-operated vibrators exist already in the form of electric toothbrushes or facial massage kits. The child should be introduced to these sensations slowly, and reactions carefully observed and recorded. If a child responds particularly strongly to vibration, then its use should be slowly increased in order to enable the child's potential for learning to be realized.

Conclusion

The use of vibration has been shown to be advantageous to the education of certain children, generally those with the greatest level of handicap. However, because of the variable nature of the response of such children to sensory input, the use of vibration should be monitored carefully. In this way too, a more extensive body of knowledge about the effects of this technique should become available.

References

Antonitis, J.J. & Barnes, G.W. (1961). Group operant behavior: On extension of individual research methodology to real life situation. *Journal of General Psychology*, **98**, 95-111.

Byrne, D.J. & Stevens, C.P. (1980). Mentally handicapped children's responses to vibro-tactile and other stimuli as evidence for the existence of a sensory hierarchy. *The Journal of the British Institute of Mental Handicap*, **8**, 96-98.

Glover, E. & Mesibov, G.B. (1978). An interest center sensory stimulation program for severely and profoundly retarded children. *Education and Training of the Mentally Retarded*, **4**, 172-177.

Goodall, E. & Corbett, J. (1982). Relationships between sensory stimulation and stereotyped behavior in severely mentally retarded and autistic children. *Journal of Mental Deficiency Research*, **26**, 163-175.

Goodall, E., Corbett, J., Murphy, G. & Callias, M. (1982). Sensory reinforcement table: an evaluation. *Mental Handicap*, **10**, 52-55.

Hogg, J. (1983). Sensory and social reinforcement of head turning in a profoundly retarded multiply handicapped child. *British Journal of Clinical Psychology*, **22**, 33-40.

Jones, C. (1980). The uses of mechanical vibration with the severely mentally handicapped. Part 2: Behavioral effects. *Journal of the British Institute of Mental Handicap*, **7**, 81-82.

Rice, H.K. & McDaniel, M.W. (1966). Operant behavior in vegetative patients. *Psychological Record*, **16**, 279-281.

Schaefer, H.M. (1960). Vibration as a reinforcer with infant children. *Journal of the Experimental Analysis of Behavior*, **3**, 160.

Stevenson, H.W. & Knights, R.M. (1961). Effect of visual reinforcement on the performance of normal and retarded children. *Perceptual & Motor Skills*, **13**, 119-126.

Verity Hobbis, Tim Williams, clinical psychologists, Mary Sheridan Unit, Borocourt Hospital, Wyford, Reading, Berkshire, 964 RJD, England.

Evaluating and Stimulating Vision in Multiply Impaired Children

R.T. Jose; A.J. Smith; K.G. Shane

Abstract: The authors describe techniques for evaluating a multiply impaired child's functional level of vision and give a sequence of vision stimulation for those children found to have vision. They stress the importance of creativity and flexibility on the part of the teacher and underscore the need for piecing together whatever functional information the child may reveal to various individuals, including parent, educator, and doctor.

When a multiply impaired, "low level" child has vision he or she is not using, this is often because it is easier for the child *not* to use it. If the child has a sensory integrative problem (information may be received from all the senses but in a kind of disconnected confusion—for example, a tickle may seem like a pain, or a quiet, calm sound may seem irritating or brash—the information being processed through the visual system may be confusing or "not processed" at all. In this instance, the child seems to be blind. Often, the child is unaware that there is any vision and needs training in how to use it. These children may be frightened, self-abusive, non-responsive, or under the effects of strong medication and, as a result, seem to be "non-visual."

Since it is difficult to obtain or understand the responses from these children, the conventional method of eliciting a response usually has no effect. In order to reach out to the child in his or her world, it is necessary to be flexible in our structure. There are many clues that the child may be inadvertently giving, and by piecing the functional information together, the educator, parent, and doctor can begin to obtain an idea of the child's visual system.

The following is a functional visual evaluation adapted from Langley and DuBose (1976).

For educators to successfully plan vision stimulation programs, they must first observe, evaluate, and record all information that indicates the child's functional level of vision. So much can be learned about the child's level of visual functioning by simply observing him or her in a variety of situations—such as in the classroom, at play, or while eating.

The purpose of this evaluation is to increase observational skills and to decrease assumptions. First, observe whether the child exhibits a change in his or her behavioral response to any stimuli, be it auditory, visual, or tactual. Then look for any indications as to whether or not the child is functioning visually. Examples of behaviors to observe are: neck and facial straining; postural changes such as head tilts; and different visual behaviors such as light gazing and flicking.

Observe the child's mobility. Does he/she move with ease and speed? Does the child exhibit smooth range of movement? Does he/she shuffle feet while walking? Does he/she walk with head down? Does the child avoid or bump into objects? If so, are they consistently on one side or below knee level, for example? As you observe, note whether the child tends to be functioning more on a visual level or mainly through other sensory modalities.

The items covered represent samples of visual sensation, visual-motor, and visual perceptual skills. To obtain a more accurate and comprehensive picture of the child's visual functioning, record more than just the presence or absence of a response. For example, when the object is presented to the child, describe the illumination of the room, the type and size of the object, and the distance from which the child sees it. If the task, distance, or position of the child is changed in any way, indicate this on the screening form. Then answer the following questions about the child's responses: Is he or she using both eyes? Does the child perform independently or require assistance? What behaviors does he or she demonstrate while responding to each evaluation item?

Pupillary response
To test whether a child's pupil responds to light, start by observing the condition of the pupil without stimulation. There are abnormal conditions such as hippus, constant small constrictions and dilations of the pupil, or fixed pupil, a pupil that will not constrict or dilate regardless of the amount of stimulation. Then direct a penlight into the child's eye from approximately 12 inches (30cm) away. Observe whether the pupil constricts, dilates, or remains the same. In general, it can be assumed that if a child's pupils constrict upon the presence of light, the child is demonstrating a reaction to light.

If the pupils are not responding to the penlight, observe the child's pupils when he or she emerges from a dark room after a period of time. A millimeter ruler, or optistick, most accurately measures change in pupil size. Try using a brighter light source, or extinguish the room light to provide increased contrast. Be sure to present the light in different fields of view, not only directly in front.

Muscle imbalance (tendency for the eyes to deviate)
Shine a penlight into the child's eyes from approximately 30 inches (76cm) away and note if the light is reflected in corresponding places in both eyes. If the light reflection in one eye is offcentered, or different from that of the other eye, this deviation should be noted. Hold the light in different places and vary the distance. Remember that with some conditions such as aniridia and leukokoria, it may be difficult to see a reflection.

Blink reflex
With fingers spread apart, move your hand toward the child's face. Be careful not to create a wind by moving your hand too quickly, because the child might be blinking in response to the wind rather than to the visual stimulus.

Different visual behaviors
Note visual behaviors, such as flicking and light gazing, which may indicate light

The information in this article was developed at the Center for the Blind/Upsal Day School for Blind Children, in Philadelphia, Pennsylvania, under HEW contract 300-76-0352 (Clinical-Educational Interaction for Enhanced Visual Functioning of the Multiply Handicapped Blind Child). Based on a paper given at the Wisconsin Workshop: Services for Deaf-Blind Persons, Madison, Wisconsin, April 30 and May 1, 1979.

projection and shadow perception. Although these behaviors are labeled socially unacceptable, they might often be the only indication that the child is using his or her vision.

Eye preference
While holding a light or small object 12-18 inches (30-45cm) in front of the child's eye, alternately cover each eye and record if the child demonstrates any behavioral changes. The child may resist having his or her better eye patched. This resistance could also be caused by tactual defensiveness. To avoid touching the eye, block the vision by holding your thumb in front of the child's pupil. If the child does or does not resist having his or her eye patched, does that necessarily indicate that one eye is preferred?

Central fields
Shine a penlight approximately 12 inches (30cm) from the child's face. Note whether the child attends to the light. Then, shine it slightly above, below, to the left and the right of his or her face. If the child demonstrates no response to the light, try either moving it in closer, blinking the light, or using a different type of color of light. If the child demonstrates a response to the light (this may be a head or eye turn), then repeat the procedure with small objects.

Peripheral fields
Position yourself behind the child and slowly bring the light into the child's field of view from above and below, and from left to right, and right to left. Record at which point the child reacts to the light. If the child responds to the light, repeat the procedure using small objects. When presenting the light or object, it is important to maintain a consistent arc or distance from the child's face. The movement and speed of the light may need to be varied with each child. Be aware that reaction may be to your arm (auditory, olfactory) rather than to the light. It may be necessary to suspend the light or object from an invisible string.

Visual field preference
Choose two identical lights or objects to which the child responds. Simultaneously, present them to the child's right and left visual fields. Record whether the child responds to both fields or demonstrates a preference for one. If the child attends to one object rather than to both, is the object or the visual field being preferred? Can the child be ignoring one field rather than not seeing it?

Tracking ability
Use lights, squeeze toys, puppets, or whatever small object will hold the child's attention. With the light or object held within the child's range of vision, move it slowly to the right, left, up, down, and circularly. Note how efficiently the child locates the light or object, whether he or she is attending to it and how long the child is able to maintain attention. This activity should be presented to the child's peripheral as well as central fields. Note whether the child is following with his or her head, eyes, or both. Comment on whether the tracking appears smooth or jerky and if the child experiences any difficulty tracking across his or her midline, and whether tracking is being done with one or both eyes.

Reaching for lights and objects
Place lights, toys, and other visually stimulating objects at various levels and directions from the child. Note whether the child turns toward and reaches for them. For children who are only capable of prone, supine, or stationary positions, place lights and objects within reach. For example, hang lights or shiny objects from the ceiling to the child's eye level.

Shifts attention
Hold two familiar lights or objects in front of the child. Shine, blink, or shake one; pause; and then repeat the actions with the second light or object. Note whether the child shifts attention. Vary the position of the lights and objects presented in the child's central and peripheral fields. Some children experiencing problems with motor coordination may need additional time to respond.

Scanning ability
Place three objects in front of the child and note whether he or she searches in a line from one object to another. Remember to place the objects within the child's best field of view. Experiment with central and peripheral fields. Remain aware that the child may need to be motivated to respond.

The last section of the evaluation involves an integration of visual and cognitive skills. When working with more severely impaired children, be aware that responses may be a result of their level of cognition rather than visual development.

Approach
With activities involving stacking cones, cylinders, puzzles, pounding benches, beads, and so forth, note if the child accurately inserts or manipulates objects. Record any overreaching or underreaching.

Observe whether the child looks for the recess or hole or tactually approaches it.

Matching
Show the child one colored block, shape, or picture and observe whether he or she is able to match it with a similar corresponding object or picture. Repeat with a variety of shapes, colors, and sizes. Observe which colors, shapes, and pictures the child matches best. Attempt to determine if the child's attention is directed to color or to configuration. Observe the distance at which the child can correctly match various objects. Note if the child is using any other senses while matching.

Ability to follow moving objects
From containers, tap or pour blocks and pellets directly in front of the child and note whether he or she looks at them as they tumble out. If there is no response, try presenting the task in other areas of the child's visual field. To diminish any auditory cues, work over felt or other sound-absorptive surfaces. Other suggested materials for this task are colored water, sand, marbles, and "Slinkys."

Imitation
With a wide felt tip pen, scribble many large circles on white paper in front of the child. Observe whether the child attempts to take the marker. Or a physical action in front of the child, then note whether he or she tries to imitate your actions.

Object-concept
Give the child a large colorful book or Peabody Picture Card. Record whether he or she bends to touch the picture, looks at it, or gives any response that indicates awareness of something on the paper. With some non-ambulatory children, look for any movement that may indicate recognition.

Object permanence
Place food or an object in one of your hands and present both hands to the child, open. Close both hands and note if the child tries to open the appropriate, or either hand.

Means-ends
Give the child a toy that has continuous action and attracts his or her attention. As the child watches, move the toy out of sight and note if the child looks for it. Replace it in front of the child and note if he or she attempts to reactivate it. If possible, use a toy that does not make any sounds (e.g., Nerf Ball). For those children who are physically incapable of reactivating the toy, look for any movement

that might indicate the child is attempting to do so. Note the response mode with which the child attempts to act on his or her environment.

Keep in mind, when working with severely impaired children, that several sessions may be necessary to complete the evaluation. A child might, for example, require more time to respond or need assistance from the evaluator in order to respond. At times during the evaluation, additional stimulation might be necessary just to motivate the child. It is important, in attempting to elicit responses, to communicate with the child on any level he or she understands.

With the aid of this information, the educator and parent begin to be aware of the child's visual functioning and the eye-care specialist is better able to adapt and interpret clinical testing. Ongoing interaction between the eye-care specialist and educator is an essential component of this program. Information gathered from the evaluation and follow-up visits is related to the child's educational program. In turn, information gathered from the child's visual functioning in the classroom is integrated with the optometric evaluation.

While some clinical data may be obtained from a responsive child within minutes, the same data may require as long as nine months with some less-responsive children. Therefore, the evaluation should be considered an ongoing process.

For a thorough diagnosis of the child's visual system, the following data should be collected: awareness of lights; acuity; presence of refractive error; binocularity; visual fields; and the confirmation of ocular health reported by previous eye-care specialists.

The starting point of the evaluation is the pupillary response, which provides an indication of visual potential. If there is no pupillary response, it should not be assumed the child has no visual potential. Instead, that child should begin a program of vision stimulation to determine if a visual response can be obtained.

For visually impaired children, the development of vision is not an automatic process. The child's visual system must be stimulated before the child can be taught how to see.

Establishing visual acuity level

In the first stage of the vision stimulation program, the educator finds a stimulus to which the child responds favorably (e.g., the sound of bells or the sensation of a vibrator), and then pairs this stimulus with the presentation of light. Gradually, the other stimulus is removed until the child responds to the light alone. Once the child's visual system has been awakened, it is easier to establish a level of visual acuity.

The acuity evaluation first involves discussions between the eye-care specialist and educator concerning questions such as: Does the child seek light, have a favorite toy or color, reach for specific objects, or use vision while traveling?

It is important to determine even the minimum stimulation to which the child seems to be responding visually, for this is the foundation of the vision stimulation program. For example, if the evaluator can determine the presence of light projection in a child, the educator can help develop this into gross form perception and object detection. This will be particularly useful in the child's mobility.

Once the child responds to light, he or she is taught to follow a moving light. The evaluator should try colored or flashing lights to help stimulate the child's interest and attention.

Progressing through the vision stimulation sequence, the child learns to attend to objects. At this level, the eye-care specialist can establish a gross acuity. For example, the evaluator holds an object in one hand, then presents both hands. The child must then locate the object by visually exploring both hands. As the child becomes accustomed to this task, the evaluator begins to stand farther away with hands spread three to four feet apart. The test distance and object size can be changed until the child's highest or best acuity level can be established.

In determining acuity, the evaluator is trying to provide the educator with the potential visual functioning of the child. The numbers attached to this diagnosis, e.g., 20/20 or 20/200, are not as important as the information that the child can see a half-inch (1.2cm) block at three feet. By knowing the size of objects and the distance at which they can be seen by the child, the teacher is better able to plan appropriate educational activities. Other recommended activities are:
• Attending and responding to an optikinetic drum;
• Picking up objects from a surface, such as a desk or the floor;
• Matching exercises with toys, utensils, and other familiar objects;
• Responding to picture cards, lighthouse symbol cards, or objects of various sizes drawn on nonreflective surfaces; and
• Responding to familiar objects viewed on a video monitor.

It is important to note that when object sizes or test distances are varied, it may be necessary to teach the child to respond to each task as if it were a new task. A lack of response may indicate a need for training and not a lack of vision.

In any case, the results of these activities are only estimates. The child should not be given the level of a 20/20 or a 20/200 acuity without investigating the implications of this label upon the child's individual educational plan.

For those children who show no indication of visual acuity, an electrodiagnostic evaluation may provide additional information to confirm a diagnosis. However, electrodiagnostic testing with low level multiply impaired children should never be used as a basis for educational judgments. In many cases, these children will not be able to attend to the test situation for even the short period of time necessary to obtain accurate information.

Refractive correction a possibility?

The next step in the optometric evaluation is to determine if a refractive correction will improve the child's acuity. To assist the evaluator in performing a retinoscopy, the teacher may create a fixation point for the child. The teacher must attract the child's attention by shining lights, holding puppets, talking or singing, or holding any favorite or familiar object.

If the child is cooperative, an ophthalmoscopy can be performed. In this case, the ophthalmoscope lens required to focus on the retina will approximate the refractive error, providing the evaluator is not accommodating or does not require a refractive correction.

It is helpful to role play with the child so he/she can become accustomed to the testing procedures before the eye-care specialist evaluation. This training should be done by educators, parents, and all others directly involved with the child.

If a retinoscopy or ophthalmoscopy cannot be obtained, the eye-care specialist may provide either a high plus or high minus spectacle correction and observe behavioral changes. The evaluator can increase or decrease the lens in small diopter steps until the child's behavior and functioning seem to be best. Extreme caution should be taken with some seizure-prone children. A high plus or minus lens may cause too much of a change in the child's visual system, and as a result may induce seizures.

The eye-care specialist should also consider using contact lenses as a diagnostic tool for those children who cannot wear spectacles.

Although some children may benefit visually from lenses, they may be so tactually defensive that they will not tolerate the spectacles. Because of this, it may be difficult to determine whether the change in behavior is due to the child's tactual defensiveness or the lens change. The educator needs to work patiently in teaching the child to wear the frames alone and then to wear both the lens and the frames.

Testing binocularity

In order to evaluate the child's binocularity, the eye-care specialist and the educator must work closely together. In the cover test, the child's eyes are alternately patched. This may reveal an eye turning in, out, up, or down. The Hirshberg test determines the posture of the binocular fields, as indicated by the reflection of a penlight shone in the child's eyes. Other binocularity tests require the child to wear red-green glasses. Then, the evaluator observes the child's behavioral response to red or green light. In addition, higher functioning children may be able to verbally respond to the colored dots of the Worth 4-Dot Test.

Patching is another method of evaluating binocularity. If the child responds negatively to being patched and demonstrates less functional visual performance, it can be hypothesized that the child's better eye is covered. However, the child's reaction may be a result of tactual defensiveness, fear, or annoyance. Also, some children may just not demonstrate a response to any stimulus and any assumption of presence or lack of binocularity may be misleading.

Testing fields

Since testing visual fields requires discrimination from the child, it is often more difficult to determine. The eye-care specialist relies heavily upon the educator's observations.

A confrontation test is one method for testing fields. Lights, toys, and food are presented from behind the child while the teacher, in front of the child, holds the child's attention and reports his or her reactions. Be aware that the child may be responding to sound or to movement. If this is the case, the object or light can be suspended from a string.

A more difficult test is to ask the child to fixate on one object while another is presented in the periphery. The child then indicates when the object comes into his or her field of view.

When objects are scattered on a surface in front of the child, he or she is asked to find all the objects, while maintaining the head in one position. If an area is consistently ignored by the child, then a field loss may be indicated.

If a lower field loss is suspected, base down prisms may be applied to the child's spectacles. Behavioral changes or increase in field activity may be observed.

Another way to confirm a suspected field loss is to occlude the area of suspected loss. If the loss is real, the child should not show a difference in functioning or behavior. If there is no loss, a behavioral change should occur.

The eye-care specialist and the educator, when combining their efforts, can achieve a common goal—an evaluation of the child's functional vision. In order to obtain a realistic estimate of the child's visual functioning, a multi-disciplinary approach—with cooperation between doctors, educators, specialists and parents—is essential.

Vision stimulation sequence

As the visual functioning of the child is understood further, the educator and family can begin to implement a program of visual stimulation.

The following sequence of vision stimulation is designed to be adapted for populations ranging from multiply impaired to those with low vision as their only handicap. Suggestions for adaptations in certain steps in the sequence will be provided to reflect individual differences.

The sequence is not intended to be a cookbook approach and if followed as such will hamper the creativity and flexibility of the teacher and the child. Of utmost importance is the consideration of the individuality of each child and his or her approach to the learning situation.

The arrangement is not hierarchical. This means that it is possible for the child to be functioning on a step further on in the sequence, without being able to perform the earlier tasks. It is recommended that each person start the sequence from the beginning. This eliminates the assumption that the child is functioning at a certain level and ensures the discovery of developmental lags, which may result in visual perceptual problems later on.

Observation

Observe the child for change in behavioral response to any stimulus. Then observe for anything that leaves a doubt as to whether or not the child is functioning

visually. Behaviors to observe are: facial straining; postural changes such as head tilts or compensatory body adjustments; and different visual behaviors such as light gazing or flicking.

Regarding gait, does the child shuffle his or her feet, walk with head down, etc.? Observe the child's mobility. Does he or she move with ease and speed? Is smooth range of movement exhibited? Does the child avoid or bump into objects? If the child bumps into objects, where are they located (e.g., head high, waist high, low lying) and is the child consistently bumping on one side more than the other? Is the child functioning more on a visual or other sensory level (e.g., groping behavior, exploration with eyes, hand, mouth)?

Awareness of any stimulus

Using any stimulus (e.g., object, light, sound, smell, temperature change), observe when child displays a consistent change in behavioral response upon presentation of the stimulus. The stimulus chosen should be one to which the child responds favorably, as it may be necessary to pair it with a visual stimulus at a later step in the sequence.

Recommendations

1) Place child in a small darkened room, where walls have been lined with aluminum foil. String Christmas lights (blinking and non-blinking) and suspend mobiles and objects that would reflect the lights, thus creating an environment of visual bombardment. If a small room is not available, position the child to face the corner of any room. Line the corner walls with aluminum foil, and suspend the above-mentioned lights and objects. If possible, darken the room for contrast.
2) Touch the child with or allow the child to touch an encased (foam rubber) vibrator. Guide and encourage the child to manipulate the vibrator.
3) Attempt stimulating any sense with a variety of experiences. Check the advisability of the use of blinking lights with some seizure-prone children. The use of sensory bombardment with every child is not always indicated. Check medical history and proceed with caution. If using tactual stimuli, consider the degree of tactual defensiveness of the individual child.

The proper position for the individual child must be investigated with occupational and physical therapists, parents, doctors and all those involved with the child before the implementation of any steps in the sequence.

Attention to any stimulus

Once a stimulus has been found to which the child seems to respond, efforts should be made to elicit a consistent response each time the stimulus is presented to the child.

Generally, with more severely involved children, there is a different "consistency" in the time interval involved in responses to stimuli (i.e., child may perseverate for long periods of time or display very short attention spans).

Pairing a light with the stimulus to which the child has responded

Each time another stimulus is presented, introduce a light source (e.g., flashlight, penlight), for as long as the child maintains attention. 1) Shake tambourine in front of light, while light source is on. When light is turned off, tambourine is still. 2) Present light source to child, while rocking child who has been positioned over a roll. When rocking ceases, turn off light source. The purpose of these activities should be to assist the child in becoming more aware of the light and to associate the positive stimulus with attention to the light.

Avoid consistently placing light source directly in front of the child, since this may not be in the child's area of functional vision. Attempt placing light at various angles.

Awareness and attention to light stimulus alone

Intermittently, shine light source alone, without pairing with the other stimulus. Note whether the child gives the same response.

Several different types of lights should be experimented with, as many children may not exhibit responses to penlights or flashlights. Placing different colored filter paper in front of the light source, using flickering or colored lights, shining lights through a translucent surface, or pairing light with any stimulus that the child consistently responds to are examples of various types of light sources and ways of presenting them.

Monitor child's response to light (e.g., turns to avoid light, pushes it away, constriction of pupils, reaches for light). Note the area of the visual field in which the child consistently responds or does not respond to lights. Light sources should be presented in all areas of the visual field.

Do not assume that there is no visual functioning if pupils do not constrict. Several conditions, such as nerve damage; hippus; fixed pupils; or some medical conditions of aniridia, may inhibit the pupillary reflex.

Attention to light stimulus alone

Gradually decrease pairing of light with other stimulus until child consistently responds to light source alone. Each time the light is presented to the child, he or she will demonstrate consistent visual attention.

In some instances, although the child may be visually attending, this might not be evident because the child's eyes do not appear to be directed towards the stimulus. This could be due to various factors such as field loss and eccentric fixation. Therefore, when observing the behavior, attention should be directed towards the consistency of ocular movement.

Localization of light source (awareness)

Light is presented in all visual fields. Note child's behavioral reaction (e.g., turns head, moves body part towards light).

A variety of lights should be used (varied color and intensity, translucent and transparent filters). Room can be darkened for heightened contrast. Vary position of child (sitting, kneeling, prone, supine, over roll) to find which best facilitates awareness of light.

Note preference for transparent or translucent colored light. Any time a non-self-contained light is used, place Plexiglas between child and light source. This reduces heat variable and prevents accidents.

Localization of light source attention

Light source is presented in all visual fields. Child is required to look at light in each position.

Note child's beginning attention span and gradually require more visual attention. Note area which child consistently ignores. This may be an indication of field deficit.

Observation of child's tracking ability

Preferred light source should be presented horizontally, vertically, obliquely, and circularly, while child tracks (follows a moving light with head, eyes, or a combination of both).

Observation of how the child tracks lights should be made (e.g., with head, eyes, combination). Are the movements smooth or jerky? Does the child lose the light at his or her midline? Does child experience difficulty following the light across the midline?

Teaching saccadic or choppy tracking

Child will visually follow light blinked on and off along a line. Pace and increase of blinking should be individually determined. Sequence of presentation of light should be horizontally, vertically, obliquely, and circularly.

When teaching these visual motor skills, observe the following sequence: (a) head movement tracking; (b) eye movement tracking; and (c) head and eye movement tracking (not necessarily in that order).

Construct a piece of cardboard with 1/2-inch (1.2cm) holes along a line (holes may be outlined). Slowly move light behind cardboard. Experiment with varied colors, transparencies, and translucencies.

Hold a xylophone at eye level with keys facing child. In the same manner as above, move light in back of the xylophone. With some children, encourage hitting the xylophone keys as light passes behind.

Teaching smooth tracking

Initially, if there is no response to tracking, it may be necessary to physically aid the child. The child's head may be moved in the direction of the light source until the child can do this independently. In order to facilitate eye movement independent of head movement, it may be necessary for the educator to hold the child's head. As the child masters this tracking skill, head and eye movement are then combined.

When teaching these visual-motor skills, observe the following sequence: a) head movement tracking; b) eye movement tracking; and c) head and eye movement tracking.

During the initial stages of tracking skills, the child's other senses should be combined (e.g., allow the child to hold the light source as it moves and give verbal cues as to the directions of the movements). Gradually, these additional sensory cues are removed and the child is required to track by visual cues alone.

Provide the child with appropriate light sources, which will encourage as much independent manipulation as possible.

Initially, to provide contrast, it may be necessary to darken the room. Be alerted to the possibility of tactual defensiveness and results of conditions such as cerebral palsy, where separation of head and eye movement may be difficult or may touch off an asymmetrical tonic neck reflex. In the above instances, and for many children with additional handicaps, correct positioning is essential in facilitating vision. Consultation with occupational and/or physical therapist is most important in this area, as incorrect positioning of the child may preclude success in stimulating his or her vision.

Awareness of whether light is on or off
Light source is presented, then blocked (with opaque material). Child should exhibit difference in behavioral response either independently or with guidance. 1) Place child next to light table (photographer's) and direct attention (verbally or by moving child's head) to the light source. Then totally block the light by placing opaque material, such as cardboard or carpet remnant, over the light. 2) Previous procedure can be followed using any non-diffuse light source such as a tensor lamp.

Attention to whether light is on or off
As light source is repeatedly presented and blocked, the child will demonstrate consistent visual attention.

Gradual decrease in size of object blocking light source
Instead of total blockage of light source, an opaque material allowing partial blockage of light is used. The size of the opaque material is then gradually reduced, allowing a continual increase in light area. 1) Use decreasing sizes of carpet remnants. Tactual reinforcement is provided by allowing the child to remove the remnant. 2) Use a variety of objects of decreasing sizes, such as cardboard, large puzzle pieces, small boxes, and dark colored cookies (this is both useful and motivating because the child is permitted to bite the cookie). He or she receives sensory reinforcement while reducing the blockage of light.

Comments
Educators should be discriminating in the use of food as a primary reinforcer for visual activity. In some instances, food reward may not be appropriate (e.g., in cases of dietary restrictions for medical reasons, or when the classroom teacher is trying to wean the child from functioning only when offered food as a reward).

Sensory reinforcement (e.g., touching carpet and eating cookie) gives the child the chance to experience objects through other modalities, which may facilitate beginning of the awareness of objects.

Note when the child begins to have difficulties locating the object; you may be testing child beyond his or her visual capability. Be aware of the minimum size of blockage of light the child is able to locate.

Gradual decrease in background illumination
Instead of higher intensity illumination, repeat the above steps while using light sources of decreasing intensity. 1) The use of a dimmer switch, or rheostat, is most effective when light table is utilized. 2) When using tensor lamp begin with 150 watt bulb, then replace with 100 W, 75 W, 60 W, 30 W, 15 W, etc. 3) Use various light sources of decreasing intensity (photographer's light, tensor light, lamp light, flashlight, then more diffuse, such as room light). 4) For some children, contrast—and thus ease of task—is facilitated if room lights are turned off.

Note level of background illumination at which child begins to experience difficulty distinguishing objects, as further decrease in illumination may be testing child beyond his or her visual capability. Be aware of the lowest intensity of illumination at which the child is still able to locate the object (blockage of light).

Generalization of the above activities over a variety of environments and with different materials
Instead of the use of one object or light source to elicit a response from the child, different classroom or environmental objects are experimented with in an effort to avoid splintering and transfer learning. 1) Use a variety of objects, not necessarily of increasing or decreasing size. Hold the objects directly in front of the light source and observe difference in child's behavioral response (e.g., directs attention toward, moves toward, reaches for, attempts to smell). 2) Begin with presenting objects in areas of lesser intensity (e.g., from well lit to dimly lit rooms, from hallway lights to outdoor environment at various times of the day and under various weather conditions. Objects chosen should not necessarily be those to which the child responds favorably (i.e., objects should be unfamiliar as well as familiar).

Attending to objects
Initially, the child may not be aware of an object the way we perceive it, as described in the preceding activities. Instead, he or she may perceive and attend to an object as a blockage of light. Attention may also be due to the characteristics of the object. At this stage, the child should be required to exhibit visual attention and not just a behavior change in response to the light. Recommendations: 1) Utilizing as many objects as possible (e.g., brightly colored, light-reflecting, multi-patterned, different sized, noise making), encourage the child to explore the objects with his or her other senses. 2) At this point, the child's observable functional field should be known, and presentation of objects should be initially directed in those areas. However, presentation of objects in other areas of the child's visual fields should be continuously explored (e.g., move object circularly, gradually increasing the circumference of the circle to cover other areas of the child's visual field). This increases the area of the child's awareness of his or her fields and encourages the child with limited fields to move his or her head. 3) Continue to vary the background contrast and illumination.

Object tracking
Object should be presented horizontally, vertically, obliquely, and circularly, while child tracks moving objects (follows with head, eyes, and a combination of both). 1) Follow the same sequence listed with tracking lights. 2) During the initial stages of tracking skills, the educator should combine the child's other senses (e.g., allow child to hold light source as it moves and give verbal cues as to the direction of the movement). 3) Emphasize a diversity in objects presented. Examples of common objects that can be used include balls, tops, wind-up toys, friction toys, bubbles, balloons, and puppets.

Factors such as difficulty crossing midline, tactual defensiveness, and nystagmus, are common conditions affecting a child's ability to track. Correct positioning and consultation with physical and occupational therapists and doctors should be sought in an effort to determine and facilitate child's overall functioning.

Movement exploration with objects
Though reaching for and moving towards lights and objects should be encouraged throughout all the preceding activities, exploring objects in space is emphasized here. 1) Suggested materials: large and small balls, moving toys, obstacle courses, etc. 2) Place child and some large objects in a confined area (e.g., large carton in which a washing machine could have been shipped). Allow child to play with objects by moving them and himself/herself in the carton. Talk to the child about the restriction of movement. 3) Repeat 2 with large objects, child, and large area; small objects, child, and large area.

Emphasis should be placed on eye/body coordination tasks. Initially, the child may need physical guidance for correct movements, as efficient eye/hand and eye/foot coordination may not necessarily be exhibited by him or her. Hand and foot movements should be directed into the child's functional field of view.

Most important is that we have confidence in our ability to teach these children. To accomplish this, it is essential that we become more flexible and that our expectations be based on the individual child, and not on our preconceived structure.

It is the responsibility of each person involved with the multiply impaired child to put aside the stereotype that these children are too "low functioning" to be able to learn, and to underscore the concept of a multi-disciplinary approach in an attempt to reach a common goal. If the child is met with labels, lower expectations, and stereotypes, the self-fulfilling prophecy will be actualized.

References

Langley, B. & DuBose, R.B. (1976). Functional vision screening for severely handicapped children. *New Outlook for the Blind,* 70(8), 346-350.

Randall T. Jose, chief, Audrey J. Smith, orientation and mobility specialist, the William Feinbloom Vision Rehabilitation Center, Eye Institute, Pennsylvania College of Optometry; Karen G. Shane, low vision coordinator-instructor, The Diocesan Human Relations Services, Orono, Maine.

Functional Vision Screening for Severely Handicapped Children

B. Langley; R. F. DuBose

Abstract: Ophthalmologists traditionally have been unable to provide teachers and parents with useful information about a severely handicapped child's functional vision. Literature concerning the assessment of vision in handicapped children is reviewed and a guide is proposed for use by teachers in evaluating the severely handicapped child's functional vision.

Severely handicapped children with some form of visual impairment are often placed in educational settings accompanied by inadequate reports giving some indication of visual classification and an unintelligible description of the specific impairment. References are repeatedly made to the difficulties involved in assessing the child's visual problems and to the hesitancy with which the ophthalmologist makes his judgment. In centers where a multidisciplinary team evaluates the child, vision experts tend to rely on the functional visual information provided by the classroom teacher or the educational diagnostician. A more practical assessment of visual functioning in severely handicapped children will therefore become available if those agents most familiar with the child's everyday use of vision actually participate in the assessment.

This paper describes some of the difficulties found in testing the visual acuity of severely handicapped children, surveys formal and informal measures used in testing visual acuity or functional vision, suggests guidelines for teachers to use in observing visual behaviors, and proposes a functional vision checklist that may be used by teachers or paraprofessionals to gain insight into how a child is using his residual vision.

Formal assessment of visual acuity

The problems inherent in determining visual acuity of multiply handicapped children have been stated by Allen (1957), Wolfe and Harvey (1959), Hoyt (1963), Sloan and Savitz (1963), Ffooks (1965), Borg and Sundmark (1967), Faye (1968), Lippman (1969), Macht (1971), and Sheridan (1973). Under the conditions im-

posed by the instruments used for testing visual acuity, low functioning children are easily distracted, lose interest in the test, fear the testing situation, fail to understand the tests, and give unreliable and inconsistent responses. Special educators and ophthalmologists have tried to find visual acuity tests that are effective with severely handicapped children, since visual impairment is frequently found with other handicapping conditions. Blackhurst and Radke (1968) found that moderately retarded children had four times as many visual impairments as the normal school population; Vernon (1969) reported that approximately 25 percent of deaf children had some form of visual impairment; and Wolf and Anderson (1973) provided evidence of visual limitations in 50 percent of cerebral palsied children.

What is visual acuity?

Wolfe and Harvey (1959) defined visual acuity as the ability to distinguish small spatial separations, or intervals, between portions of the visual field. Since it depends upon the ability of the eye to resolve a given visual angle, acuity is greater the closer together are two points that can be distinguished. Wolfe and Harvey distinguished sensory from visual acuity as an individual's reaction to low-keyed sensory data of mild duration and extent. Lippman (1969) suggested that sensory impressions developmentally advance from discriminative and perceptual stages to a conceptual stage.

Sheridan (1970) segmented acuity into two separate processes which are particularly relevant to multiply handicapped children: *seeing* and *looking*. Described as a physiological process dependent upon intact visual mechanisms, *seeing* is "the

reception of mobile and static patterns of light, shade, and hue by the eye and transmission of this information to the central nervous system" (Sheridan, 1973). Primarily a psychological process, *looking* combines perceptual and conceptual operations to attend to visual stimuli with purposeful interpretation of their meaning.

As the child's awareness of his world increases, so does his ability to distinguish visually and to respond to more abstract forms of stimuli through gradual refinement of his acuity to its mature state. Sheridan (1973) believes that by 12 months a child has a visual acuity comparable to adult vision, although it is not efficiently developed. A child of kindergarten age should be able to attend to an object for at least 20 seconds, pursue a moving target in all directions with a minimum of head movement, and localize different visual stimuli within the environment (Banus, 1971).

The majority of multiply handicapped children with significant visual deficiencies retain some functional vision and do see. However, their limited experiential and cognitive repertoires—essential to the integration of sensation into meaningful stimuli—prevent them from looking.

Formal tests and procedures

The formal tests that offer the most promising information about the extent of visual functioning of multiply handicapped children are Sheridan's Stycar Vision Tests and Koehler's New York Flashcard Vision Test (Faye, 1968). These tests were developed specifically for use with handicapped children and to assess near as well as distant vision.

Lippman (1969) found the Stycar to be the most reliable test in screening visual acuity of preschool children. Although Sheridan devised a distant screening chart consisting of only nine capital block letters chosen on the basis of simple vertical and horizontal lines (L H T), the circle (O), the cross (X), the part square (U), the triangle (A), and the part-triangle (V), her Miniature Toys Test and Rolling Balls Test (subtests in the Stycar battery) are in fact more useful for evaluating vision in multiply handicapped children.

The Minature Toys Test was developed for use with severely handicapped children who were unable either to match letters or name and match colored pictures of common objects placed individually on cards. After experimenting with numerous toys, Sheridan found the most effective ones to be a car, plane, doll, chair, knife, fork, and spoon, all 2″ high; a larger knife and spoon 3¼″ high; and a doll 5″ high. She found that children as young as 21 months successfully matched the objects and that their interest in the task lasted for its duration.

Designed particularly for use with children from six to 30 months, the Rolling Balls Test consists of a series of graded balls projected a distance of 20 feet. The child is required to retrieve them one by one after they have been rolled horizontally across his line of vision.

The New York Flashcard Vision Test was developed out of a need for assessing the visual acuity of multiply handicapped children, visually handicapped preschool children, and the nonreader of any age (Faye, 1968). Only three symbols (heart, house, and umbrella) make up the test. They are presented one at a time on 12 reversible 4″ x 5″ flashcards. Snellen acuity notation is printed on every card, three symbols for each acuity level from "200" characters to "10." As long as they are consistent, children may verbally or manually label symbols anything they like or, if unable to express themselves, can point to large matching symbols. Average children of 27 months consistently attended and responded appropriately to the three symbols, and Faye successfully screened trainable mentally retarded children with the cards. The test is administered in the conventional method of acuity testing, except that the test distance is ten feet or less and notations can be converted to the 20-foot reading.

Unsuitable Tests
Other formal measures of visual acuity have required skills not in the repertoire of multiply handicapped children. Sloan and Savitz (1963) identified two major forms of visual acuity tests, those based on indicating directions and those requiring identification of pictures.

In reviewing tests based on indicating directions, Sheridan (1973) felt that the Snellen E, the Sjorgen-Hand Test, and Landolt's Broken Rings included three major factors that significantly influenced the low functioning child's ability to perform adequately on them. Because multiply handicapped, as well as preschool children, have difficulty in coping with diagonals, they responded only to figures pointing up, down, left, or right. Directionality also complicates the assessment of multiply handicapped children, as they confuse left and right and, although they

may perceive laterality, they experience confusion in duplicating the position of the symbols. Because the patterns presented are constant, no opportunity is available to observe the child's ability to discriminate differences in configuration (Sheridan, 1973; Ffooks, 1965).

Picture identification tests have been most frequently employed in testing handicapped populations, though numerous adapted procedures have been necessary. Osterberg (1965) specified three requirements to bear in mind in the selection and development of pictorial visual acuity charts: 1) optometric principles must be adhered to as closely as possible; 2) objects must belong to the child's world of ideas; and 3) presentations of pictures must be adapted to the child's demands for recognition of pictures greatly variant from adults' needs. Other authors (Allen, 1957; Wolfe & Harvey, 1959; Hoyt, 1963; Faye, 1968; and Sheridan, 1973) have stressed the importance of using pictures of objects within the child's experiential repertoire. General criticisms of picture charts were that the pictures inaccurately projected angles at a nodal point corresponding to the highly accepted Snellen E symbol and required personal experience and ability to recall labels. More specific concerns have been expressed by Sloan and Savitz (1963), Borg and Sundmark (1967), and Ffooks (1965). Sloan and Savitz (1963) and Ffooks (1965) stated that picture tests were too dependent on psychological interpretations of figures before they could be understood and recognized by children.

Informal testing of visual acuity
Adaptations of formal tests have included deleting items; projecting them onto large screens; manipulating three-dimensional response materials; converting response forms into puzzles; altering the type of figure, outline, silhouette, background, or color of the target and response figure; and applying operant technology (Courtney & Heath, 1971; Macht, 1971). Although numerous tests have been developed and adapted with handicapped children in mind, none have proved satisfactory for use with this population unless administered through some form of operant procedure.

Employing an operant approach, Courtney and Heath (1971) trained and evaluated color vision in 39 trainable and 71 educable mentally retarded children using the AO HRR Color Vision Tester to determine the percentage of color blindness

among the population of mentally retarded individuals. They found the AO HRR effective, as it offered four training and six testing plates graded for both type and severity of color blindness. The test proved to be highly motivating, required no verbal responses, no ability to read conventional numbers, and no need for the coordination essential for tracing paths. Training the children to take the color form of the test was accomplished through a black-and-white adaptation of the colored symbols O, X, and △. Identical forms were painted on slabs hinged to a box which dispensed M&M's whenever a correct response was given. Most children required about five minutes of training, but the authors succeeded in testing one 12-year-old Mongoloid child with an IQ of 35 after 40 minutes of training. No difference was found in the prevalence of color blindness among mentally retarded individuals and that of normal individuals reported in the literature.

Macht (1971) applied operant technology to obtain a subjective measure of visual acuity in five mentally retarded children between five and seven years of age. He included in his subject population two adults of normal intellectual and visual functioning to verify his results. Through the use of a specially constructed wheel displaying two stimulus Snellen Illiterate E's, one at the top and the other at the bottom of the wheel, and a table containing a response mechanism, Macht not only devised a way to evoke responses to the Snellen Illiterate E Chart, but also included an elaborate training system. The children were placed at the table 20 feet from the wheel and were trained to respond by pushing the response lever to the upright E, as opposed to the E which inverted as the wheel turned. Subjects were reinforced with M&M's and small candies for appropriate responses. The initial training E was larger than 20/200, but for the actual testing the 20/200, 20/100, 20/70, 20/50, 20/40, 20/30, and 20/20 E's were utilized. Obtaining significant successful results that correlated with the adults' responses, Macht attributed children's previous failures to respond to the Snellen E and other visual acuity tests to procedural inadequacies rather than to the presence or absence of some quality in the child.

Macht and Courtney, with their promising results, offered the field of visual assessment valuable implications for successful application of tests that had previously proved ineffective with multiply handicapped children. Teachers cognizant of how children functionally use their vision can give ophthalmologists information that is helpful in determining visual capacities. Assessing functional vision in the severely handicapped child is a first step in planning educational programs relevant to his or her needs.

Informal teacher-oriented visual screening

Informal teacher-oriented visual screening procedures can effectively obtain important, practical information regarding what a child sees and how well he sees it. Although informal, the evaluation should be carried out systematically. Establishing a working rapport with the child, the setting, and stimulus materials is of primary importance. With particularly young children, it may be necessary to hold and rock or sing to them for several minutes to quiet them. Sharing a manipulative toy often helps the evaluator to gain the confidence of an older child. The setting should be small, uncluttered, and quiet. Working with the child on the floor, where the evaluator has easy access to both the child and materials, facilitates administration of stimulus materials, puts the child and evaluator on the same level, and prevents attempts to leave a table, slip from a chair, or push materials from the table. Multiply handicapped children are more responsive to higher motivating materials, although in this assessment they must be limited in sound components to insure that the child is attending visually rather than aurally.

Suggested materials for eliciting visual behaviors outlined in the checklist are brightly colored soft rubber squeak toys with the speaker removed (this toy can be squeezed to produce action but the sound is eliminated), a penlight or small flashlight, fluorescent rubber toys containing lights, and mechanical toys having flints producing sparks when operated. Especially motivating for severely handicapped children are rattles encasing moving parts; large and small spinning tops and easily rolled cars; fluorescently colored inch-cubed blocks; small candies or cereals such as M&M's, Fruit Loops, cake decorating items; and roly-poly action toys. Other suggested materials are a small box, paper and brightly colored magic markers; plastic pegs and board; brightly colored, textured books with thick pages; large beads; stacking cones; a primary puzzle with approximately three pieces; multicolored counting bears;

shape-sorting chips or parquetry blocks; simple pictures in duplicate glued to small index cards; or commerically produced pictures and duplicates of different colored toys for matching.

The first stage of the visual assessment should be to observe the child for immediately obvious visual abnormalities and behaviors indicating deficient vision. Primary questions to be answered should focus on the presence or absence of basic visual responses, and the types of visual stimuli (light, movement, color) to which the child attends. Observing not only the manner and direction in which the child reacts to visual stimuli, but also the distance and size of objects eliciting the most consistent response, provides insight into the positioning of specific materials useful in obtaining maximum visual attention. Equally important is the assessment of the child's ability to integrate visual stimuli with cognitive and motor processing skills to perform discrimination, association, figure-ground, and eye-hand coordination activities. Simple techniques for use in assessing five aspects of visual function are given below. Figure 1 suggests checklists a teacher may use for recording information about a multiply handicapped child's performance.

Techniques for functional vision screening

I. Presence and nature of the visual response

a. Direct a penlight into the child's eyes from 12″ away and observe whether the pupils constrict, then dilate when the light is removed. Be sure to observe his eyes before shining the light as blind children often exhibit hippus, a continual constricting and dilating of the pupil.

b. Assessing a tendency of the eyes to deviate can be done by flashing a beam from a penlight into the child's eyes from 30 inches away. If the light is reflected simultaneously in the middle of each pupil, no deviation is present. If the reflection is centered on one pupil but off-center in the other, some form of muscle imbalance is indicated.

c. Place the child on his back and kneel behind his head. Pass your hand across his eyes, pause and repeat. A blinking reflex indicates some light perception and possibly some object perception.

d. Assess the child's perception of light using a penlight. From 12 inches or closer, flash the light and note whether he attends to it. The light should be flashed slightly

above, below, to the left, and right of the child's face to determine the range of visual field. Note whether he fails to attend to the light in any plane.

e. Sitting behind the child, bring the light slowly into his right, then his left visual field. Note at which point he turns to look at the light. He should notice it when it is directly in line with the lateral portion of the eye.

f. Present the child with play objects of equal interest simultaneously in the right and left visual fields and gesture for him to touch them; switch their positions and repeat. Observe whether the child attends to a toy in only one position rather than both.

g. While holding a motivating toy 12 inches to 18 inches in front of the child's eyes, alternately cover each eye. Observe whether he resists having one or both eyes covered or if he remains indifferent to the covering. Children having limited or no vision in an eye will not mind having that eye covered but will strongly resist covering of the functional eye.

II. Reaction to visual stimuli

a. Observe the child for any inappropriate visual behaviors such as light flicking with fingers or objects or eye poking.

b. Evaluate the child's ability to localize, track, and scan by holding puppets, small squeeze toys, or penlights within the child's range of vision. Move them slowly from left to right, up and down, and in oblique angles. Note whether he locates an object efficiently and attends for at least 20 seconds.

c. Place toys at all levels and in all directions and watch to see if he turns and reaches for them. These items should be interspersed throughout the evaluation to maintain interest in looking.

d. Note whether the child is able to shift his attention by holding two toys of equal interest approximately one foot apart in front of the child. Shake one, pause, then shake the other. Observe whether he shifts his gaze to the other toy.

e. Observe his ability to scan by placing three objects in front of him and watch to see if he shifts his attention from one toy to the next in line.

III. Distance and size of objects and pictures

a. While interacting with the child, scatter small pegs or candies ¼ inch in diameter, inch-cubed blocks, counting bears, or shape chips around the child and encourage him to find them. Note the distance at which he most consistently attends to variously sized objects.

I. Presence and nature of the visual response

a. Pupillary reaction: __present __absent __R __L
b. Muscle imbalance: __present __absent __R __L
c. Blink reflex: __present __absent __R __L
d. Visual field loss: __present __absent __R __L
e. Peripheral field loss: __present __absent __R __L
f. Visual field preference: __present __absent __R __L
g. Eye preference: __present __absent __R __L

II. Reaction to visual stimuli

a. Inappropriate visual behaviors: __present __absent
b. Tracking ability: __present __absent
   __light __objects: __vertical __circular
   __horizontal __oblique
c. Reaches for toys: __present __absent
   __in front of him __to his right __to his left
   __above eye level __below eye level
d. Shifts attention: __present __absent
   __both sides __one side __R __L
e. Scanning ability: __present __absent

III. Distance and size of objects and pictures

a. Locates dropped toy: __present __absent __distance
   __peg or candy __inch-cubed blocks __shape chips
b. Small toy observed: __present __absent __distance
c. Large toy observed: __present __absent __distance
d. Objects matched: __present __absent __distance
   __large toys __distance
   __small toys __distance

IV. Integration of visual and cognitive processing

a. Visual pursuit: __present __absent
b. Causality: __present __absent
c. Object permanence: __present __absent
d. Object concept: __present __absent
e. Means-ends: __present __absent

V. Integration of visual and motor processing

a. Approach:
   1. pegs: __visual __tactual reach: __O __U
   2. stacking cone: __visual __tactual reach: __O __U
   3. puzzles: __visual __tactual reach: __O __U
   4. pounding bench: __visual __tactual reach: __O __U
   5. beads: __visual __tactual reach: __O __U
b. Matching:
   1. colored blocks:
      __matches __does not match __near distance __far distance
   2. shapes:
      __matches __does not match __near distance __far distance
   3. pictures:
      __matches __does not match __near distance __far distance

Figure 1. Information checklist.

b. Project large (6″ to 8″ in diameter) and small (2″ to 3″ in diameter) toys to the left, right, and forward from the child and observe how far they travel before he looks away or ceases in his efforts to retrieve them.

c. Using a set of toys that duplicate, except for color, those used in b, have the child match his objects with yours as you display them singly. Begin at 10 feet for large and 5 feet for small objects. Obtain the maximum distance at which the child sees the objects without straining by moving backwards or forwards in 2-foot intervals until he consistently matches four or five objects.

IV. Integration of visual and cognitive processing

a. Tap or pour blocks and pellets from containers in front of the child. Note whether he looks at them as they tumble before him.

b. Scribble large circles with a magic marker on white paper in front of the child. Note whether he watches or attempts to take the marker.

c. Give the child M&M's to hold, help him place them in a small box and shake them around. Take the box from the child and quickly remove the candies. Watch to see if he looks for the candies when you return the box.

d. Give him a large colorful book to look at. Note whether he bends to look at the pictures or pats them.

e. Give the child a toy which has continuous action and attracts his attention. As he watches, push the toy out of his sight and note if he looks for the toy. Replace it before him without the motion and observe whether he attempts to reactivate it.

V. Integration of visual and motor processing

a. On activities involving the pegs, stacking cone, puzzles, pounding bench, and beads, watch to see if he directly inserts or applies pieces, overreaches (O), or underreaches (U). Does he look for the recess and the hole or does he only tactually approach them?

b. When shown one colored block, shape, or 2-inch picture at a time, can he match it, given only two choices? Watch to see which colors, shapes, and pictures he matches and if he attends to color or configuration. Observe the distance from the materials at which he works, then have him match them at a far distance. Note the farthest distance at which he correctly matches each.

Summary

Traditional tests of visual functioning and acuity have lacked the impetus essential for assessing children with multiple impairments. Although operant measures have been successful in eliciting behaviors required to respond to these tests, Sheridan and Koehler have offered the most promising formal tests for this population. Until the use of the New York Flashcard Vision Test and the Stycar Vision Test is more widespread, the task of visual assessment remains primarily with the teacher. Obtaining even a gross indication of the child's functional visual field—a preferred eye, distance at which he most efficiently works with variously sized objects, and the level of complexity of the visual stimuli that the child successfully interprets—provides the teacher with basic information needed to design an educational program relevant to the child's visual and developmental needs.

References

Allen, H.F. (1957). Testing of visual acuity in preschool children: Norms, variables, and a new picture test. *Pediatrics, 19,* 1093-1100.

Banus, B.S. (1971). *The developmental therapist.* Thorofare, NJ: Charles B. Slack.

Blackhurst, R. & Radke, E. (1968). Vision screening procedures used with mentally retarded children—a second report. *Sight Saving Review, 38,* 84-88.

Bord, G. & Sundmark, U. (1967). A comparative study of visual acuity tests for children. *Acta Ophthalmologica,* **45,** 105-113.

Courtney, G.R. & Heath, G.G. (1971). Color vision deficiency in the mentally retarded: Prevalence and a method of evaluation. *American Journal of Mental Deficiency,* **76,** 48-52.

Faye, E.E. (1968). A new visual acuity test for partially-sighted non-readers. *Journal of Pediatric Ophthalmology,* **5,** 210-212.

Ffooks, O. (1965). Vision test for children: Use of symbols. *British Journal of Ophthalmology,* **49,** 312-314.

Gorman, J.J., Cogan, D.G., & Gellis, S.S. (1957). An apparatus for grading the visual acuity of infants on the basis of optokinetic nystagmus. *Pediatrics,* **19,** 1088-1092.

Hoyt, W.F. (1963). Neuro-ophthalmologic examination of infants and children. *International Ophthalmology Clinics,* **3,** 757-775.

Lippman, O. (1969). Vision of young children. *Archives of Ophthalmology,* **81,** 763-767.

Macht, J. (1971). Operant measurement of subjective visual acuity in non-verbal children. *Journal of Applied Behavior Analysis,* **4,** 23-26.

Osterberg, G. (1965). A Danish pictorial sight-test chart. *American Journal of Ophthalmology,* **59,** 1120-1123.

Sheridan, M.D. (1973). *Manual for the Stycar Vision Tests.* Windsor, Ontario: NFER.

Sloan, A.E. & Savitz, R.A. (1963). Vision screening. *International Ophthalmology Clinics,* **3,** 815-831.

Vernon, M. (1969). Multiply handicapped deaf children: Medical, educational, and psychological considerations. Washington, DC: Council for Exceptional Children Monograph.

Wolf, J.M. & Anderson, R.M. (1973). *The multiply handicapped child.* Springfield, IL: Charles C Thomas.

Wolfe, W. & Harvey, J. (1959). The evaluation and development of techniques for testing the visual and auditory acuity of TMR children. *Eric document 002 802.* Austin, TX: College of Education, Texas University.

Beth Langley, M.A., educational diagnostician; Rebecca F. DuBose, Ph.D., associate professor, Faculty of Special Education, Model Vision Project, George Peabody College for Teachers, Nashville, Tennessee.

IDENTITIES

Recognition of one's own needs, from the level of maintaining personal comfort through engaging in social interaction, is vital in establishing a stable sense of self. The two articles included here provide two perspectives on the process of respecting one's own importance.

Behavioral Treatment of Aggression and Self-Injury in Developmentally Disabled, Visually Handicapped Students

J.K. Luiselli; R.L. Michaud

Abstract: Management problems are often encountered among developmentally disabled populations. The authors describe behavior modification treatment procedures that were applied by direct-care staff in a residential school to control severe aggression and self-injury in two developmentally disabled, visually handicapped students. In one case, the aggressive and self-injurious behaviors of an 11-year-old with vision and hearing deficits were reduced by positive-practice overcorrection. In the other, a blind adolescent's self-injurious behavior was eliminated by a combination of restitutional overcorrection, verbal command, and response-immobilization techniques. The practicality of applying behavioral treatment procedures in educational settings for visually handicapped students is discussed.

Educating children who have both sensory and intellectual impairments is a complex endeavor. The development of effective remedial education is even more complicated when these children present severe management problems. Of the many maladaptive behaviors exhibited by developmentally disabled students, aggression and self-injury create the most difficult management problems. The most debilitating effect of these behaviors is that they produce physical damage. These behaviors also are incompatible with learning, interfere with a teacher's ability to carry out meaningful instruction, and introduce anxiety and tension into the teaching environment. Finally, aggressive and self-injurious students are frequently avoided by others, which limits the interpersonal contact that might improve their academic and social functioning.

Neuroleptic drugs and mechanical restraints such as camisoles are often used to manage severe problem behaviors (Mulick & Schroeder, 1980). Although these approaches may reduce the frequency of such behaviors, environmental factors that might be maintaining the unwanted behaviors are ignored. In addition, neuroleptic drugs have deleterious side effects such as tardive dyskinesia,

hypoactivity, and tremor. Prolonged restraint leads to bone decalcification and reduced range of motion. Finally, both approaches inhibit adaptive, prosocial behaviors (Marholin, Touchette, & Stewart, 1979; Rojahn, Schroeder, & Mulick, 1980).

Therapeutically, the most desirable strategy for managing severe problem behaviors is to teach significant others, such as teachers and parents, how to program the interpersonal environment in a manner that encourages adaptive skills and discourages maladaptive acts. Treatment programs based on behavior modification principles provide such a strategy (Wilson & O'Leary, 1980). Since advocates of behavioral approaches view management problems as stemming from improper learning, intervention focuses on re-arranging environmental contingencies to foster more appropriate responses. Consequently, behavioral methods are particularly well suited to educational settings because procedures can be integrated into teaching activities, which enable direct-care staff to apply treatment on a day-to-day basis within a student's natural environment.

The purpose of the current research was to evaluate the implementation of behavioral treatment procedures with two

developmentally disabled, visually handicapped students who were aggressive and self-injurious. Both students attended the same private residential school for individuals with visual and hearing deficits. All treatment and data collection were carried out by special education personnel who were trained to implement the program through a behavioral consultation model that has proved to be effective in the treatment of visually impaired children in residential schools (Luiselli, 1981a).

Andrew

Andrew was an 11-year-old male with a hereditary 18th-chromosomal abnormality, a cataract in one eye and a surgically repaired retinal detachment in the other, arrested hydrocephalus, with scoliosis, which was being corrected by a Milwaukee brace. He spoke only in brief phrases and could carry out simple oral instructions. Overall, Andrew's functional skills fell within the moderate range of mental retardation. In addition to his skill deficits, he was aggressive toward others and hit himself in the face and head. His aggression interfered greatly with student and adult interactions; his self-injurious behavior was a serious problem because of the possibility that he would dislodge surgically implanted aural tubes and damage his repaired retina.

The treatment program was implemented in Andrew's classroom, where one teacher and a full-time aide provided instruction in language, academic, self-care, and recreation skills. Andrew attended class from 9:00 A.M. to 3:00 P.M. Monday through Friday, with two other students.

Target behaviors and data collection

Two behaviors were targeted for intervention: *self-injury* was defined as any time Andrew hit his face or head with one or both hands; *aggression* was defined as any incident of hitting, pinching, biting, or pulling the hair of an adult or another child. The teacher recorded the frequency of these behaviors daily on a precoded data sheet. To assess reliability, the junior author observed classroom activities regularly for 30 to 60 minutes (observations occurred at random times during baseline and treatment days). After each observation period, the frequency of the behaviors recorded by the teacher and the psychologist were compared, and reliability was computed by dividing the smaller recorded frequency by the larger one and multiplying by 100. Because of the discrete nature of the target behaviors, reliability estimates were 100 percent on all occasions.

Procedures

Procedures were implemented in an ABAB reversal design—baseline, treatment, baseline, and treatment (Hersen & Barlow, 1976).

During the first baseline phase (3 days), teaching staff were instructed to respond to Andrew's target behaviors in their customary manner. Typically, this consisted of either reprimanding or redirecting Andrew orally to respond in an alternative manner. Thus, during baseline, target behaviors were recorded in the absence of formal intervention.

During the overcorrection phase (23 days), Andrew was required to participate in five minutes of functional arm-movement training (Foxx & Azrin, 1973) whenever he exhibited aggressive or self-injurious behavior. Contingent upon a target behavior, the teaching staff said "no," seated Andrew in a chair, and instructed him to clasp his hands behind his back, then hold his hands at head level by bending his elbows and holding his upper arms perpendicular to his body. (Andrew was not asked to extend his arms fully because of restrictions imposed by his back brace.) Each position was maintained for 10 seconds. If Andrew did not comply with an instruction within two seconds, he was moved physically through the respective response using the minimal amount of guidance required. Although Andrew never performed the overcorrection movements by himself, he did not resist manual guidance. Because adult attention was judged to be a potent reinforcer for Andrew, staff members were also instructed to increase their attention to Andrew when he engaged in appropriate behaviors such as working at manipulative tasks and playing with peers.

Baseline conditions were then reinstated for two days. During this phase, the target behaviors were recorded but the staff discontinued the overcorrection procedure.

When overcorrection was introduced once again for 12 days, direct-care staff in Andrew's residential living unit also applied the intervention. Therefore, during this phase, treatment was in effect seven days per week across all settings.

After 39 days of baseline and treatment, the treatment procedures continued but data collections were terminated. One month later, the target behaviors were recorded each day for one school week. During this follow-up period, treatment remained in effect.

Results

The results of Andrew's treatment are presented in Figure 1, which shows the rate of aggressive and self-injurious behaviors recorded per hour in the classroom. During the first baseline phase, target behaviors occurred at an average rate of 4.2 per hour. When overcorrection was introduced, the behaviors decreased steadily to an average hourly rate of only .80. During the second baseline phase, target behaviors remained low on the first day, then increased dramatically to an average of 1.9 per hour on the second day. When overcorrection was reinstated, the target behaviors dropped to an average rate of .48 per hour. One month later, the effects of treatment were maintained at an average of .36 per hour.

Ted

Ted was a severely retarded 19-year-old who had been blind since birth because of maternal rubella. On performance testing for blind children, his functional skills fell in the 12- to 27-month range. Ted's expressive language was limited to one-word statements and occasional short phrases. Without physical assistance, Ted was unable to respond to most instructions or perform independent self-care skills such as washing, dressing, and grooming. In addition to these deficits, Ted presented several behavior problems, including vocal disruptiveness, noncompliance, and arm-biting (the target behavior).

At a previous treatment facility, attempts to reduce Ted's arm-biting through reinforcement and punishment techniques were unsuccessful. Ted also had been placed on a daily regimen of Chlor-promaxine (Thorazine) to control his behavior, but this too was ineffective. Ted was finally dismissed from the treatment facility because of his unmanageable self-injurious behavior.

Ted received training in a classroom staffed by a teacher and an aide and in his living unit, which was supervised by two child-care workers. Two other blind, developmentally disabled students shared Ted's classroom. Training activities in the classroom and living unit consisted of language, prevocational, self-care, housekeeping, and recreational skills.

Target behavior and data collection

Ted's target behavior of arm-biting consisted of placing his arm in his mouth and biting down forcefully. This behavior had produced continuous dermal abrasion and numerous open sores on both arms. Frequency of arm-biting was recorded on a precoded data sheet by Ted's teacher and by child-care workers from 9:00 A.M. to 9:00 P.M., Monday through Friday. To assess reliability, the senior author periodically recorded data with the staff in a simultaneous but independent manner

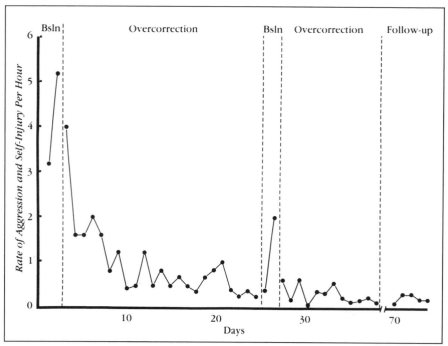

Figure 1. Rate of Andrew's aggressive and self-injurious behaviors recorded per hour during the baseline and treatment phases and follow-up.

for 30 minutes to 2 hours. Reliability was computed in the manner described earlier. Throughout the study, reliability averaged 87 percent.

Procedures

Procedures were implemented in an AB design: one baseline and one treatment phase. During baseline (five weeks), staff were instructed to record the incidents of arm-biting they observed and respond to it in their customary manner. Typically, they responded by reprimanding Ted; occcasionally, they removed him from activities until he stopped biting. They also tried to praise him as much as possible for responding appropriately during training and for using his hands properly.

The treatment program (15 weeks) consisted of antecedent and consequence control procedures. As a consequence of arm-biting, Ted received restitutional overcorrection training (Foxx & Azrin, 1972). Contingent upon an arm bite, the staff members said, "When you bite your arm, you must care for yourself." Then they led Ted to a designated bathroom, placed him in front of a sink, and guided him physically through the following sequence of behaviors:

1. Picks up a container of antiseptic cleanser and squeezes a small amount into a plastic bowl.
2. Returns the container.
3. Picks up a premoistened napkin.
4. Dips the napkin into the antiseptic solution.
5. Applies the napkin to the bitten areas and pats the area lightly 10 times.
6. Repeats steps 4 and 5 twice.
7. Places the used napkin in an empty container.

Throughout overcorrection, the trainer guided each response using the minimal amount of physical assistance required. Although we anticipated that Ted might resist such guidance, he was compliant during all applications of overcorrection. Each overcorrection episode lasted approximately five minutes.

The antecedent control feature of intervention consisted of interrupting a chain of responses that appeared to be a precursor to arm-biting. During baseline, we observed that before biting his arm, Ted often seemed agitated: he made a whining sound, flailed his arms, and banged his ankles against each other. Because this agitation seemed to be unrelated to the context of a particular activity, intervention was aimed at stopping the agitation

with the expectation that this might obviate subsequent biting. The procedure consisted of the following steps: A staff member said, "Ted, calm down" whenever Ted displayed 10 consecutive seconds of agitation. If the agitation had not ceased within 10 seconds of the command, a back-up procedure was used—Ted was placed in a chair located in a designated area; the staff member sat behind him and held his arms to his sides until his agitation had ceased for one minute. When this criterion was achieved, Ted was allowed to stand up and return to his previous activity. As they had done during baseline, the staff continued to praise Ted for appropriate outer-directed behavior and the absence of arm-biting.

Results

The results are presented in Figure 2. The top panel shows the average number of arm-biting incidents recorded weekly during baseline, treatment, and follow-up phases. During baseline, Ted bit his arm an average of 9.8 times each week. When treatment was in effect, the frequency of this behavior was reduced to an average of 2.3 incidents per week. During the

four-month follow-up period, only four instances of arm-biting occurred, and during the final five weeks, none occurred.

The bottom panel in Figure 2 displays the average number of verbal commands and applications of immobilization that occurred weekly. During treatment, an average of 3.3 commands were required each week. During follow-up, an average of only .75 were required. The back-up immobilization procedure was required infrequently: on an average, 1.2 times per week during treatment and only three times during the 16-week follow-up period.

Discussion

The goal of these studies was to provide direct-care personnel with efficient management programs to control aggressive and self-injurious behaviors among developmentally disabled, visually handicapped students. According to the results, the treatment programs were successful in reducing the target behaviors to manageable levels. The procedures were integrated easily into each student's daily routine, and staff members had no difficulties

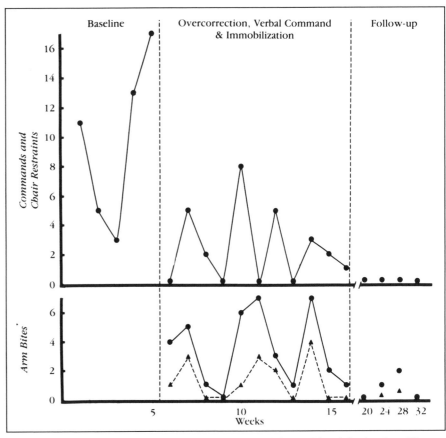

Figure 2. Number of Ted's arm-biting incidents and the residential school staff's verbal commands and applications of immobilization recorded each week. Data during follow-up represent the average frequencies per week during each four-week period.

implementing them. In fact, the reduced frequency of the target behaviors achieved by the staff made it easier to carry out instructional activities with the students.

With Andrew, who had visual and auditory deficits, positive practice overcorrection was effective in controlling both his aggressive and self-injurious behaviors. Although overcorrection has been used before with visually handicapped clients (Kelly & Drabman, 1977; Luiselli & Rice, 1982), to our knowledge, ours is the first case in which the procedure has been used to treat the combined problems of aggression and self-injury in a child with multiple sensory impairments. Note, however, that the desirable effects obtained with Andrew cannot be attributed unequivocally to the overcorrection procedure alone because the teaching staff also increased their attention to his positive behaviors. Therefore, reinforcement of alternative responses may have been operating in conjuction with overcorrection. Perhaps the most parsimonious way to view these results is to regard Andrew's treatment as an "overcorrection package" composed of positive practice and reinforcement—a combination that Foxx and Azrin (1973) suggested is the most desirable format for programming overcorrection.

With Ted, overcorrection was also used in a combined treatment package. One component of this package was the manipulation of antecedent events. The fact that this procedure was included is noteworthy because approximately 90 percent of behavioral treatment programs for self-injury rely on consequence-control techniques (Schroeder, Mulick, & Rojahn, 1980). Since multiple factors influence the etiology and maintenance of self-injurious behavior (Carr, 1977), focusing exclusively on the consequences of such behavior may limit the effectiveness of treatment. Although the results with Ted must be regarded as preliminary in nature, the verbal command did appear to interrupt a cycle of agitated behavior that typically resulted in arm-biting. For example, during the final week of baseline, Ted bit his arm 17 times. During the first week of treatment, the verbal command "No" was stated on four occasions and arm-biting was not observed. Since Ted was not exposed to the overcorrection contingency during the first week of treatment, the reduction in arm-biting could not be attributed to that component of the treatment package. Unfortunately, the frequency of Ted's agitated behavior

was not assessed during baseline. Such data would have shown whether the verbal command procedure led to a reduction of both agitation and arm-biting.

In their review of research methodology with visually impaired individuals, Van Hasselt and Hersen (1981) stated: "The potential utility of single-case experimental designs is yet to be fully realized by clinicians and researchers who work with visually impaired individuals." Our research included two variants of single-case designs. In Ted's case, procedures were evaluated using a simple AB design, which enables one to demonstrate that treatment gains are *correlated* with intervention. One cannot draw unequivocal conclusions, however, since the influence of factors other than treatment cannot be ruled out (Hersen & Barlow, 1976).

Methodologically, stronger inferences regarding treatment are possible with the reversal design (ABAB) that was used with Andrew. The purpose of this strategy is to show that behavior improves each time the treatment is introduced and deteriorates each time it is withdrawn, thereby demonstrating functional control of independent variables. However, such a design must be tailored to the target behaviors assessed. For example, with Andrew, only two-day baseline phases were evaluated and, in both phases, response rates were unstable. In most cases, greater stability of responding over a longer period is desirable before preceding with intervention. We chose short baseline phases because Andrew's target behaviors increased in the absence of treatment. From a clinical perspective, applying intervention after an unstable baseline is generally recognized as acceptable if the instability reflects an increase in a seriously maladaptive behavior (Hersen & Barlow, 1976). Although extending the baseline phases would have been desirable methodologically, the consultant and staff viewed the clear increases in Andrew's striking himself during the two baseline periods as justifying intervention.

As a whole, the results support our earlier work on the application of behavioral treatment programs to control severe management problems among visually handicapped children and adolescents (Luiselli, 1981a, 1982b; Luiselli & Greenidge, 1982; Luiselli, Myles, & Littman-Quinn, 1982). But most important, the results indicate that effective treatment programs can be developed and carried out on a day-to-day basis by people who interact regularly

with the student; i.e., the student does not have to be removed from the educational setting to receive specialized treatment. Using direct-care staff also expands the effectiveness of treatment because behavior control is not restricted to only a few change agents. The major effect of such intervention, of course, is to overcome problems that interfere with effective instruction, thereby creating a functional learning environment.

References

Carr, E.G. (1977). The motivation of self-injurious behavior. *Psychological Bulletin,* **84,** 800–816.

Foxx, R.M. & Azrin, N.H. (1972). Restitution: A method of eliminating aggressive-disruptive behavior of retarded and brain-damaged patients. *Behavior Research & Therapy,* **10,** 15–20.

Hersen, M. & Barlow, D.H. (1976). *Single case experimental designs: Strategies for studying behavior change.* New York: Pergamon.

Kelly, J.A. & Drabman, R.S. (1977). Generalizing response suppression of self-injurious behavior through an overcorrection punishment procedure. *Behavior Therapy,* **8,** 468–472.

Luiselli, J.K. (1981a). Evaluation of a response-contingent immobilization procedure for the classroom management of self-stimulation in developmentally disabled children. *Behavior Research of Severe Developmental Disabilities,* **2,** 67–78.

Luiselli, J.K. (1981b). Consultation in the residential treatment of visually impaired children. *Journal of Visual Impairment & Blindness,* **75,** 353–358.

Luiselli, J.K. & Greenidge, A. (1982). Behavioral treatment of high rate aggression in a rubella child. *Journal of Behavior Therapy & Experimental Psychiatry,* **13,** 152–157.

Luiselli, J.K., Myles, E., & Littman-Quinn, J. (1982). Treatment of severe aggressive and destructive behaviors in a rubella child using reinforcement and response-contingent time-out. *Applied Research in Mental Retardation,* **4,** 65–78.

Luiselli, J.K. & Rice, D.M. (1982). Assessing the education and suppressive effects of brief positive practice. *Education & Treatment of Children,* in press.

Marholin II, D., Touchette, P.E., & Stewart, R.M. (1979). Withdrawal of chronic chlorpromazine medication: An experimental analysis. *Journal of Applied Behavioral Analysis,* **12,** 159–171.

Mulick, J.A. & Schroeder, S.R. (1980). Research relating to the management of antisocial behavior in mentally retarded persons. *Psychological Record,* **30,** 397–417.

Rojahn, J., Schroeder, S.R., & Mulick, J.A. (1980). Ecological assessment of self-protective devices in three profoundly retarded adults. *Journal of Autism &*

Developmental Disorders, 10, 59–66.

Schroeder, S.R., Mulick, J.A., & Rojahn, J. (1980). The behavior definition, taxonomy, epidemiology, and ecology of self-injurious behavior. *Journal of Autism & Developmental Disorders, 10,* 417–432.

Van Hasselt, V.B. & Hersen, M. (1981). Applications of single case designs to research with visually impaired individuals. *Journal of Visual Impairment & Blindness, 75,* 359–362.

Wilson, G.T. & O'Leary, K.D. (1980). *Principles of behavior therapy.* Englewood Cliffs, NJ: Prentice-Hall.

James K. Luiselli, Ed.D.; Ronald L. Michaud, Ph.D., consulting psychologists, Behavioral and Educational Resource Associates, 275 Old Bedford Road, Concord, MA 01742.

On Gaining Independence as a Deaf-Blind Person

R.J. Macdonald

To the best of my knowledge, I was born with normal sight and hearing, but when I was three years old my parents noticed that I had difficulty in identifying people. A visit to the doctor disclosed that I was legally blind. To this day, no one knows what caused my vision problem: One doctor thought perhaps lead poisoning, while another thought it was a birth defect. A third doctor mentioned the possibility of Cogan's syndrome. In any case, the eye condition I have is known as optic atrophy, a deterioration of the optic nerve, and I am also deaf. I would like to share some of my personal experiences in learning to live independently at home, at work, and in the community.

When I was halfway through my second-grade year, I was transferred from a local public school to a special sight-saving class in another public school. Two years later, in January 1951, I was transferred again, to the Perkins School for the Blind.

While attending public school, I did not think of myself as being "different" from the other children. I played the same games they did, rode a bicycle as they did, and I enjoyed participating in athletics of all kinds, especially team sports. Because of my limited vision, I was never outstanding in any sport, yet I was almost always good enough so that the other children could not ignore me. At Perkins, however, things were different. I had trouble making friends, and I found it difficult to take pride in my sports activities; after all, my success had been at a "special" school. I think that at that time I was subconsciously ashamed of being blind.

Shortly after enrolling at Perkins, my teachers reported that I was not hearing everything that was going on in class. They said I was "not paying attention." I remember that it was always very important to me—although I never bothered to consider why—that I sit at the front of the classroom. I assumed that this was so that I could see the teacher better, but I now think I was subconsciously trying to adjust to the fact, as yet unknown to me, that I was losing my hearing.

I attended Perkins for nearly 12 years. By the time I was a sophomore in high school, I could no longer hear a classroom discussion, although I could usually understand what was said in a one-to-one conversation. My hearing was tested regularly, but I was always told that there was nothing wrong, that I could hear if I only wanted to badly enough. Later, when I was in college, I was sent to a psychiatrist, who even tried hypnosis and sodium pentathol in an effort to find out why I did not want to hear. I felt very frustrated, very guilty that I was not trying to hear, yet at the same time I did not know how to try any harder.

I graduated from Perkins in 1961, without any idea of what I wanted to do in the future. When the summer passed and I still had no plans, I was invited to return to Perkins for a postgraduate year. Because my grades were not consistently good, I had never been encouraged to consider college. However, near the end of this postgraduate year, the guidance counselor at Perkins suggested that I take the college entrance examination to see how I would do. I doubt if anyone expected much, but when I earned a school-record score on the mathematics portion of the examination, it was decided that I should go on to college.

I enrolled at Saint Anselm's College in Manchester, New Hampshire, in September of 1962, with the intention of majoring in mathematics. I was the first handicapped student the school had ever had; they were not really prepared for the experience but were willing to give it a try. Since I could not hear the lectures or see what was going on in the classroom, I usually did not attend classes; I read the books and took the examinations, and was satisfied if I did not fail. However, I was unable to obtain my mathematics books in braille and this created a serious problem for me. After two years, I changed my major from mathematics to philosophy. I chose philosophy because only one book was required for each class, and I could usually have the book transcribed into braille in

time for class. In fact, most of my college courses were chosen on the basis of which books were available in braille.

Although I did not know it at the time, my parents made many sacrifices in order to give me every possible opportunity. While I was in college, they remortgaged our home in order to pay for my braille books. My father learned braille himself and he and other relatives typed materials in large-type print for me to use in my school work.

In order to compensate for the restrictions—some real, some imagined—on my ability to participate in real-life situations, I spent my spare time reading, with a passion that has endured to the present day. As my decreasing hearing provided a growing obstacle to the development of good skills in the English language, my constant reading helped me achieve reasonably good skills in spelling, writing and self-expression, as well as language comprehension.

Another activity that gave me great pleasure was chess. I found it to be an effective way to make friends and to compete on an equal basis with my opponent without my hearing and vision problems posing an obstacle. I soon began playing correspondence games with people from all over the world. In addition, chess gave me my first opportunity to travel when I became a member of the United States team competing in the Chess Olympics for the Blind, in England in 1968 and in Yugoslavia in 1972.

After graduating from college in 1967 with unexceptional grades, I spent a year at home. I kept occupied with my correspondence chess, reading, and following local sports, but at the same time I felt very frustrated at not being employed. I kept asking my rehabilitation counselor to find me a job—any job. Finally, in late 1968, he put me to work in a sheltered workshop, a factory where all of the other workers were mentally retarded.

I thought about this job quite a bit. It was not that I thought I was any better than anyone else, but I wondered why I had spent five difficult years earning a college education, only to work sorting nails into little boxes and putting labels on them. I did not know what I could do, but I did feel I could do more than that. I quit that job after six weeks, determined somehow to reach out for something better.

A year later, in January 1970, I was accepted for training at a small school that specialized in training blind people as computer programmers. After completing this training in October of that year, I set about finding a job for myself. Shortly thereafter, I was hired by the United States Department of Labor as a computer programmer, and I have been working for the Labor Department for the past 13 years. My present title is computer specialist, a position that combines the duties of a senior computer programmer and a systems analyst.

Adulthood/independence

During my first four years of college, I lived in a dormitory on campus, and rarely left campus except to go home on weekends. As my final year of college approached, I wanted to learn to be more independent. I went to live in an apartment some four miles from campus, and took a bus to school each day. Many different buses stopped near my home, and I could neither see the sign on the bus nor hear the answer to a question if I asked if it were the correct bus. I would take the first bus that came, and if it left the familiar route I would get off and walk the rest of the way. By allowing extra time for the trip, I was never late for appointments.

Another important skill I developed was that of exploring the area in which I lived. I would spend time walking up and down the streets, learning the location of stores, studying which streets had the most traffic and where the safest crossings were located. I have never received mobility training and I can rarely see traffic lights, but I found that if I studied the traffic, and where and how other people crossed the streets, I had little difficulty in crossing streets myself.

I would also spend a lot of time at the nearby market, walking up and down the aisles to learn and remember where the various foods were located. I had enough sight to read the labels on food packages if I held them close to my eye and used a powerful magnifying glass. It took me somewhat longer to do my shopping than it would for the average person, but I was doing it myself, and that was what counted.

This technique of exploring, observing, remembering, and learning proved to be very important to me when I started working for the federal government, and I still use it successfully today. Even when I am staying for only one night in a hotel, it is important to me to explore a bit in order to feel comfortable in the environment—to learn where the ice machine is located, where the reception desk is, and

so on. If I happen to have someone with me who will tell me where these things are located, it is a big help, but I can do it myself when necessary.

By the time I joined the Department of Labor, I could no longer understand any speech. I could still hear some sounds, as I can even today, but I could not understand what the sounds were in most cases, nor locate the direction from which they came. Because of this, the only way in which I could communicate with others at work was to have them write printed notes to me, using a heavy felt marker. This was a very cumbersome method of communication, and few people were willing to spend much time doing it. My supervisor had to use this method in order to give me work assignments, but other than this there was very little communication with my co-workers.

This lack of effective communication was a very serious problem: I still had a lot to learn about my work, yet few people had the time or patience to spend with me to help me learn. It took me perhaps two years of frustration and difficult adjustment before I was able to produce work of a quality comparable to that of my co-workers. I am very thankful for the patience shown by my supervisor; in those early days, I do not think he had a very high opinion of my work, but he gave me the chance to prove my worth.

If I had little in the way of social interaction at work, I had even less at home. I had few friends who lived nearby, and making new friends was very difficult because of the communication problem. However, several of the friends I had made through correspondence chess were blind people who lived in the Washington area, and as time went on I was able to meet them and get to know them better. They, in turn, introduced me to other blind people in the area. We would get together every once in a while, usually for dinner in a restaurant. Communication was slow, through braille notes, but we generally had a good time, and these opportunities for interacting with others socially were of great importance to me.

I did not meet very many young women interested in going out with me on dates, but I did meet some, and this also opened a new door for me in my slowly expanding social life. I had a good job, which gave me enough income to be able to afford to take young women out to fancy restaurants, and after a slow start the opportunities for dates became more frequent. I think that, subconsciously, I was trying

to "buy" dates by using the appeal of a fine restaurant or exotic entertainment. Gradually, however, I developed more and more confidence in myself as a person, and became less dependent on money in developing an active social life.

My work, too, had improved to the point where I felt confident that I was doing at least as well as my co-workers. In 1974, I was presented with an award for quality service to the Department of Labor, and I was even assigned, for a time, to supervise the work of other employees. The growing sense of achievement in my work and the confidence I was developing in my social life combined to make me want to reach out for something new. I began to think of the possibility of attending graduate school in order to be trained to work with others. I had the idea, as yet vague, that perhaps if I could earn a master's degree, I could work in training others to become computer programmers.

As a first tentative step in this direction, I went to see an ear specialist to have my hearing tested. This was the first time I had ever gone to a doctor on my own, the first time a doctor ever reported directly to me rather than to my parents or my counselor. The doctor told me that I had an 85-decibel sensori-neural hearing loss or, in plain English, that I was profoundly deaf. As it was explained to me, there was nothing physically wrong with my ears, but the nerves in the inner ear that transmit the messages to the brain were damaged, and there was nothing that could be done about it. Hearing aids, he said, would probably not be of much help to me.

I have read quite a bit about the trauma many people face when they become deaf, but in my case the emotion I most remember is relief. I *knew* that, no matter how hard I tried, I could not understand what people were saying to me, and it was a profound relief to me to know that there was a valid explanation for the problem. The doctor who tested my hearing suggested that, since both my vision and hearing impairments could be traced to nerve problems, they could be related and traceable to the same cause.

The next step for me was to try to improve my communication skills, and toward this end I took a course at Gallaudet College in manual communication. Essentially, I was taught how to communicate using the American One-Hand Manual Alphabet, also known as "Fingerspelling," and some basic American Sign Language. I followed both methods by placing my hands over the other person's hands and following by sense of touch, since I did not have enough sight to follow visually.

I applied for graduate study at several colleges, and in late 1975 received word that I had been accepted by the California State University at Northridge, although I would be on academic probation because my undergraduate grade-point average was considered low. I was given a leave of absence from my work, and moved to California in January of 1976.

I found the adjustment to graduate school both difficult and stimulating. On the one hand, I had been out of school for nearly nine years, and I had never studied at the graduate level. On the other hand, I had more support that I had ever dreamed possible. I had two interpreters attend each class, and they would change places every 20 minutes so as not to get tired. I also had a note-taker in each class, a person who would take written notes that would later either be typed in large-type print or transcribed into braille. Since I had constant contact with the interpreter's hands, I could *feel* the enthusiasm, encouragement, and caring that these young people were putting into their work—and it was all to help me do well in school. It was the old team spirit again—I just *had* to do well so as not to let these people down. It was perhaps the greatest experience of my life to know that, despite being both deaf and blind, I was being given almost equal access to learning opportunities that were challenging, stimulating, rewarding, and useful.

The program at Northridge was a very strenuous one. Yet I felt that for the first time I was being given almost equal access to learning opportunities; my classmates, all of them with normal sight and most with normal hearing, had the same overwhelming schedule I had. When I received my Master of Arts degree in Educational Administration in August 1977, I had earned the only perfect 4.0 grade-point average in my class.

After graduating from Northridge, I returned to my former position with the Department of Labor. A month later, while attending the first Helen Keller World Conference on Services to Deaf-Blind Persons in New York City, I met a young Japanese-American woman from Hawaii named Eleanor Moriyasu. "Ele" was working at that time as a rehabilitation coun-selor with deaf-blind clients in California. A romance quickly developed, but the courtship was anything but simple, since we lived 3,000 miles apart. However, during the next nine months, Ele came to visit me in Washington twice, and I used up all of my vacation time and most of my savings to visit her in California seven times. We were married in August of 1978.

Adjusting to married life has posed challenges for Ele and me. In order to ensure that I can travel to work and throughout the city alone, we have always chosen living quarters that are within walking distance of accessible public transportation. I try to maintain as much independence as possible, and we share household work. For example, I take care of all our finances, do much of the grocery shopping, cut the grass, and do laundry and all the heavy chores around the house. Ele does the cooking, driving, and shopping for clothes, and when necessary she acts as my interpreter. Also, when a difficult situation comes up, such as an argument with a clerk in a store, Ele prefers to interpret for me and let me handle the situation.

During the summer of 1978, I was "lent" by the Department of Labor to the California State Department of Rehabilitation to develop a program to train deaf-blind people as computer programmers. The program was eventually located at Ohlone Community College in Fremont, not far from San Francisco. The basic philosophy of the Ohlone program was to give deaf-blind persons whatever was needed in the way of support services — interpreters, note-takers, books in braille or large-type print— in order to enable them to make their own decisions and do things for themselves. For example, we provided each student with assistance in researching what housing was available in the Fremont area, and with an interpreter and transportation to go looking for an apartment, but the students had to do their own looking and make the decision for themselves.

We had one student at Ohlone who was totally blind and had no useful hearing or speech. He came from a sheltered background, and had never had mobility training. Within a few weeks, he was able to take a bus from his home, change to another bus in the city center, and walk from the bus stop to his classes on the Ohlone campus, all without assistance from others. His pride in accomplishing this also gave him the courage to reach out for greater achievements.

At the end of 1981, the Ohlone program was terminated as a formal program because of funding cutbacks. Five deaf-blind students had successfully completed their training, and three of them had been successfully placed in entry-level jobs. The other two graduates, although unable to find work immediately, were continuing the search on their own after the close of the program, and eight deaf-blind students remained at Ohlone to complete their studies.

In June of 1981, I was elected president of the American Association of the Deaf-Blind, and this has meant a lot of work for me during my hours away from my regular job. The AADB has about 500 members at present, about half of them deaf-blind people and the other half made up of parents, professionals, and others involved with deaf-blind people. We have our own quarterly magazine, which is published in both braille and large-type print, and we have annual conventions that give deaf-blind people a chance to meet each other, learn new things, and have a good time together. Ongoing projects include the development of an electronic communication device for use in face-to-face and telephone communication, plans for a group home, and training programs to prepare professionals to work with deaf-blind people. Someday, we hope to have our own home office, with a paid staff that would provide direct services to deaf-blind people.

Deaf-blind people have come a long way in recent years. We have shown that we can make valuable contributions to our families, our friends, and our communities. Success is very possible, but it takes determined effort on the part of the deaf-blind person, encouragement and support from family members, and a positive, creative attitude on the part of professionals who work with deaf-blind people. As Helen Keller once put it, "Whilst they were saying amongst themselves, 'it cannot be done,' it was done."

Roderick J. Macdonald, president, American Association of the Deaf-Blind, Inc., 805 Easley Street, Silver Spring, MD 20910.

EXCURSIONS

Movement and the decision-making skills which accompany travel are emphasized in the following articles. Several exemplary programs are highlighted, and creative, individualized approaches are suggested.

Physically Handicapped Blind People: Adaptive Mobility Techniques

C.L. Coleman; R.F. Weinstock

Abstract: This article describes adaptive techniques used to evaluate and teach mobility to the physically handicapped blind individual, with emphasis on users of wheelchairs and walkers. We stress the importance of working closely with physical therapists and/or other rehabilitation professionals involved with the client to jointly determine the most suitable orthopedic devices. The use of electronic travel aids is discussed, and a system designed by the authors to mount the Mowat Sensor to a walker is described.

Traditional university orientation and mobility programs touch briefly on strategies for working with physically handicapped blind persons, but little has been written within the orientation and mobility field on resources or adaptive techniques for working with these people. The Nevil Institute for Rehabilitation and Service, a multiservice agency serving the blind in Philadelphia, received funds in October 1980 to operate a Center for Independent Living, with the target population being multiply handicapped blind people, including those who, for a variety of reasons, use wheelchairs, walkers, quad canes, or other mobility aids.

Over the past two and a half years, we have worked with a number of physically handicapped blind adults, and through our experience have compiled some suggested methods for adapting a standard orientation and mobility curriculum to meet the needs of this population. This article is an effort to share some of these adaptations, so that other instructors will have more information with which to begin.

Before adapting traditional blind mobility techniques to this population, it is necessary to gain a better understanding of the techniques used and problems encountered by nonvisually impaired physically disabled people in their movement through the environment. A number of resources are available that explain basic physical therapy principles and travel techniques (Weinstock, 1982). Additional information may be obtained by contacting rehabilitation hospitals, physical therapy associations, or consumer groups of the disabled.

We have found that the establishment of a good working relationship with the referring physician, physiatrist, and/or physical therapist, if the client has had previous rehabilitation, is critical to the development of a comprehensive mobility rehabilitation plan. By opening the lines of communication, the mobility instructor can obtain additional information on the client's physical condition and prognosis. It is equally important to increase the knowledge of the other professionals involved concerning the capabilities of blind individuals so that they do not limit a client's mobility goals on the basis of the client's visual problems. Input by the orientation and mobility instructor can also influence the choice of the orthopedic device prescribed.

Evaluation

The goal of any orientation and mobility evaluation is to develop a plan for teaching based on a client's medical and ophthalmological history, current levels of functioning, travel goals, and motivation. This plan is appropriate for evaluating the physically handicapped blind as well as blind individuals who do not have additional handicaps. (Included would be evaluation of functional vision, conceptual development, learning style, spatial awareness, memory, and use of remaining senses.)

Development of realistic travel goals

The results of the functional vision evaluation with the physically handicapped blind have great impact on the development of realistic travel goals. Certain factors should be taken into account to determine whether a person can travel in familiar places only, or is able to expand to unfamiliar areas. If a client does not have enough usable vision to detect drop-offs, questions must be raised concerning the client's ability to travel in unfamiliar environments. If this same client can utilize visual clues like railings or poles, or tactual clues such as end-of-building line, or textural changes in walking surfaces, he or she may be able to travel in familiar areas using a long cane in conjunction with a wheelchair. Persons using walkers would have more difficulty, even in familiar areas, as they would not have the advantage of the extension the long cane provides.

Those able to detect drop-offs under all lighting conditions at a distance sufficient to react safely may be able to travel in unfamiliar areas without the use of a long cane. An individual in a wheelchair must have adequate time to stop the chair, either by applying the brakes or by planting the feet on the ground, taking into account the rate of speed at which the wheelchair is moving. The momentum built up in a chair, even at slow speeds, necessitates the perception of a drop-off at a distance greater than if the individual were walking. If because of a field loss the individual can, with proper scanning, detect drop-offs from a distance but is unable to see them within close range, a cane should be used to confirm depth and curb location.

When doing a functional vision evaluation for a person who is unable to walk any distance, the instructor may consider having the person sit in a wheelchair. This will permit the evaluation to be performed in a wider variety of environments and lighting conditions.

Wheelchair evaluation

Evaluation of physically disabled blind persons must include taking a careful look at the orthopedic device they are or will be using to see if it is the most practical and suitable based on their travel goals and capabilities.

Ideally, the physical therapist should consult with an orientation and mobility specialist during the course of the evaluation of a blind client to receive input regarding potential travel abilities. At this time, an orientation and mobility evaluation should be done that includes an evaluation of functional vision, concept development, learning style, spatial awareness, memory, and sensory development. In order to maximize a client's travel potential, it is most important to get a clear understanding of how to integrate blindness skills with any orthopedic training and devices to be prescribed. The team approach should be ongoing so that upon discharge to the orientation and mobility specialist the correct orthopedic device(s) will have been dispensed.

As stated earlier, input from the orientation and mobility instructor can influence the choice of the orthopedic device prescribed. Take, for example, the client in a wheelchair. If it has been determined through the functional vision evaluation that the client will need to use a long cane, there are several factors the physical therapist should be made aware of before deciding which type of wheelchair to prescribe. With a standard wheelchair, use of the cane in one hand makes it extremely difficult to travel a straight line and control the direction of the chair. In order to go straight, one must turn both wheels equally or the chair will begin to go in circles. If a person has good use of his foot or feet to help in propulsion, this may aid somewhat in straight-line travel; however, this method can be slow and quite awkward.

One option to consider is the one-arm drive chair, which is designed to allow the user to steer and make turns using only one hand. Two wheels are mounted on one side of the chair; when they are turned simultaneously they propel the chair forward in a straight line. As a rule, this chair is given to people with severe weakness on one side, and so it may not automatically be considered for a blind client. Once aware of this option, the physical therapist should evaluate hand and arm strength and coordination, as this chair is heavier and may be more difficult to maneuver than the standard chair. The physical therapist and orientation and mobility specialist should jointly determine which hand will propel the chair and which will manipulate the cane.

Electric wheelchair

An electric wheelchair should be considered for those clients who have poor arm strength and cannot use a standard or one-arm drive chair, have poor endurance, or have travel goals and abilities that require them to travel longer distances over a variety of terrain. Because a visually impaired client needs more time to react to sensory stimuli, it is important when ordering the electric wheelchair to request that the operating speeds be lowered if possible.

The disadvantage of electric wheelchairs should be noted. An electrically powered chair is heavier and bulkier than other models and in most cases cannot be folded because of the battery and controls. Therefore, while easier to operate, it is awkward to transport in a car or by other means of transportation. It also requires a greater amount of maintenance. In addition, the joystick that operates the movement of the chair must be moved exactly straight ahead in order for the chair to move in a straight line. If it is pushed even slightly to the left or right, the chair will move in that direction. For the wheelchair traveler without vision this may be a problem. Lastly, cost must be taken into account. These wheelchairs generally cost around $3,000, and funding may be difficult to obtain.

Electronic travel aids

The use of electronic travel aids (ETAs) may greatly enhance the travel capabilities of blind persons who are nonambulatory. Advance warning of obstacles becomes very important with this population. Persons using walkers or crutches to ambulate may easily lose their balance and fall upon contacting an obstacle in their path. In addition, both these persons and wheelchair users would have difficulty going around obstacles once contacted. The ability to receive advance warning regarding an obstacle in one's path would allow the individual to alter the path of travel before making contact and thus avoid the problems mentioned above. The use of an ETA would allow both groups to travel with more ease and safety throughout the environment.

During the course of the evaluation, the client's ability to benefit from any of the electronic devices currently available

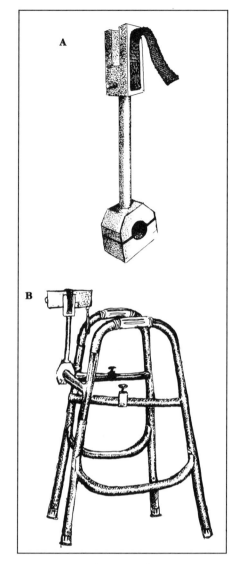

Figure 1. (A) Close-up of Mowat Sensor Holder, (B) Mowat Sensor mounted on walker.

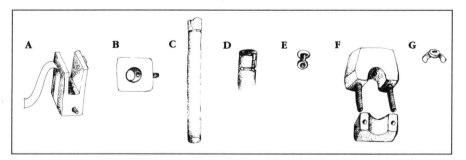

Figure 2. (A) Top piece: Insert Velcro piece inside. Glue Velcro to bottom of Mowat. Mowat is inserted and secured with Velcro strap. This piece is made of aluminum. (1) Screw with spring-loaded detent mechanism allows Mowat to be turned and locked into position. (B) Bottom view of top piece with spring-loaded pin inserted. Hole is drilled to allow insertion of steel rod. (C) Stainless-steel rod is inserted into top piece. (D) Close-up of top of rod: Guides are cut and stops drilled. Spring-loaded pin will stop at 90-degree angles and straight ahead. (E) Bottom piece: aluminum. Stainless-steel rod is inserted; held in place with a set screw (tightened with Allen wrench). Countersunk holes (threaded) hold set screw. (F) Cut out to fit walker or wheelchair. (G) Wingnuts secure to walker or wheelchair.

Box 1. Adaptations of indoor techniques.

Wheelchairs

I. Sighted guide technique
  A. Basic sighted guide
    1. Guide wheelchair, providing information about the route as necessary
    2. Alternately, guide gives verbal directions while walking beside as client wheels him- or herself
    3. Client should use seat belt whenever possible
    4. Client needs to educate guide regarding appropriate information required
      a. Making transfers to chairs, cars, etc.
      b. Appropriate use of brakes
      c. How to fold chair
      d. Operational features and accessories for wheelchair
  B. Negotiating doorways
    1. Push doors
      a. Guide wheelchair up to door
      b. If door isn't too heavy, footrests can push door open
      c. Client holds door open with appropriate hand
      d. Guide wheels through
      e. In certain situations, going through backwards may be more efficient
    2. Pull doors
      a. If client has sufficient hand and arm strength, client pulls door and holds until just before door jamb
      b. Guide wheels through, holding door with side of body
      c. If client is unable to assist with door, go through backwards
  C. Negotiating steps
    1. Two helpers should be used whenever possible
    2. Up steps
      a. Roll wheelchair backwards until large wheels are resting against riser of first step
      b. Tilt chair back until it is balanced
      c. The guide at the rear is on the second step
      d. Guide in front holds chair frame on a nondetachable part
      e. Joint effort of lift and roll, one step at a time
    3. Down steps
      a. Should never be attempted alone unless guide is *sure* he can control the chair and the weight of the client
      b. Tilt chair backwards to balance point
      c. Guide in front goes down to third step before chair is rolled to edge of steps
      d. Front guide holds chair frame securely
      e. Joint effort of letting large wheels roll over edge; reposition after each step
  D. Negotiating curbs
    1. Up curb
      a. Tilt chair and move forward until front wheels pass over top of curb and rear wheels contact curb
      b. Lower front of chair, with guide moving forward as close as possible before lifting
      c. Guide leans forward and lifts/rolls the chair up and over the curb
    2. Down curb
      a. Tip chair backwards
      b. Lower chair gently down curb, making sure both rear wheels contact pavement at the same time
      c. Alternately, turn chair around and lower back wheels onto pavement

II. Trailing
  A. Maintain contact with wall by one of the following methods
    1. Wheel parallel to wall and check position by reaching out and touching wall
    2. Attach "curb feelers" to wheels
    3. Use ETA to trail wall and detect openings
III. Turns
  A. Evaluate ability to turn with orthopedic device
    1. Depending on arm strength, may have to make several turns to complete a 90-degree turn, or may complete turn with one movement of chair
    2. Various ways to turn chair include
      a. Using both hands: one hand goes forward and one goes back
      b. Hand on side to which you are turning moves backwards, other wheel is held steady
      c. Combine use of feet with (a) or (b) above
IV. Straight-line travel
  A. Align with parallel or perpendicular wall to establish line of direction
  B. Teach proprioceptive/kinesthetic awareness of movement straight ahead
  C. Evaluate arm strength/weakness to determine if client is continually off to one side
  D. If possible, the client should use feet to help propel chair
  E. Use of ETAs to parallel wall

Walkers

I. Sighted guide technique
  A. Basic sighted guide
    1. Guide walks nearby giving verbal directions
      a. Closeness of guide depends on client's degree of balance
      b. Broken pavement may require guide to be close for "hands on" assistance with balance
    2. Develop consistent terminology, i.e., "sharp left," "angle to left," etc.
    3. Clients need to educate guide regarding appropriate information required
  B. Negotiating doorways
    1. Guide should hold door
      a. Pull door—client goes through first
      b. Push door—guide goes through first
  C. Negotiating steps
    1. Walker cannot be used on steps
    2. Client may have preferred method
      a. Use of railing plus guide
      b. Use of both hands on railing
      c. Use of quad cane and railing
    3. Railings should ideally be on side with weak leg
    4. When going up more than one flight, choice of railing may depend on which railing continues around landing
    5. Up steps
      a. Guide informs client of upcoming steps
      b. Client finds bottom riser with front legs of walker
      c. Finds railing
      d. Guide is positioned behind client, taking walker up the steps; returns it to the client at top of landing
      e. Steps up with good leg first, followed by bad leg on same step. Repeat until landing is reached

(Continued on next page)

6. Down steps
   a. Guide informs client of upcoming steps
   b. Client slowly inches forward, extends foot beyond walker to locate step edge
   c. Brings other foot forward to step edge
   d. Reaches for railing—railing should be on side of strong arm to support full weight
   e. Guide is positioned in front, facing client, carries walker and returns it to client on landing
   f. Steps down with bad leg first, followed by good leg on same step
D. Negotiating curbs
   1. Up curb
      a. Guide informs client of upcoming curb
      b. Detect curb with front legs of walker
      c. Walk up to edge of curb
      d. Lift walker above curb
      e. Step up with good leg, follow with bad leg
      f. Guide may steady walker if client has balance problem
   2. Down curb
      a. Guide informs client of down curb
      b. Client slowly inches forward, extends foot beyond walker to check for edge of curb
      c. Bring other foot forward to curb edge; front legs of walker should not be directly at edge
      d. Lower walker to street level
      e. Step down with bad leg, followed by good leg

II. Trailing
   A. Maintain contact with wall by one of the following methods
      1. Slide side legs of walker along wall
      2. Walk parallel to wall by touching wall with back of hand following each step forward; walker is several inches away from wall
      3. Attach "curb feeler" to side of walker
      4. Use ETA to trail wall and detect openings
III. Turns
   A. Evaluate individual's ability to turn with orthopedic device
      1. May have to make several small turns to make 90-degree turn
      2. Combining small turns may make accuracy more difficult
   B. Teach proprioceptive/kinesthetic awareness of turns
IV. Straight-line travel
   A. Align with parallel or perpendicular wall to establish line of direction
   B. Teach proprioceptive/kinesthetic awareness of movement straight ahead
   C. Stress importance of moving both arms equidistant out in front, rather than moving them at an angle
      1. Difficult skill to acquire as moving walker at even a slight angle can cause client to continue following that direction
   D. Look at type of balance problem or weakness to determine if client is continually off to one side
   E. Use of echodetection to stay away from wall
   F. Use of ETAs to parallel wall

should be ascertained. Farmer (1980) discusses criteria for selecting suitable candidates for ETAs and describes advantages and disadvantages of each. He includes a training format for the use of the Lindsay Russell Pathsounder for nonambulatory persons.

The Pathsounder has been the ETA of choice in the past for persons using orthopedic devices. The device does not require extensive training and gives advance warning about obstacles. Since the Pathsounder is hung around the neck, the user's hands are free. The disadvantage of using this device is the need to turn the body or wheelchair in order to use it for paralleling or scanning the environment.

More recently, the Mowat Sensor has been used as a supplementary mobility aid for people using orthopedic devices. As with the Pathsounder, this device does not require extensive training, gives advance warning about obstacles, helps to locate doorways, and aids in straight-line travel through the use of paralleling. One of the problems with this device is that it is

designed to be handheld. A system for mounting the Mowat on a wheelchair with a gooseneck extension centered in front is discussed by Morrissette, Goodrich, and Hennessey (1981). While the gooseneck mounting may have been successful for a wheelchair user, the same does not hold true for use with a walker. In attempting to mount the Mowat on a walker using a gooseneck attachment, we found that the movement of the walker jolted the gooseneck, which in turn changed the position of the Mowat, providing the user with unreliable information. We therefore attempted to devise an alternate mounting system. The system devised allowed the user to lock the Mowat in three positions: forward, for obstacle detection; and at 90-degree angles to the left or right for paralleling and detecting door openings (Figures 1 and 2).

The Sonicguide™ is another ETA that could be used by a physically handicapped blind individual in that it allows the person to scan the environment while leaving the hands free to maneuver the

wheelchair or walker. However, when considering this device, one must look at the types of environment in which the client will be traveling. The interpretation of complex signals requires a great deal of training, and the Sonicguide™ may, in fact, provide more sensory information than is necessary for a user traveling in familiar areas only.

One of the primary concerns for a blind traveler using a wheelchair or walker is the detection of drop-offs. None of the three ETAs mentioned above addresses this issue. The Step Sensor, manufactured by Nurion, has been evaluated at Hines Veterans Administration Hospital and is now in production. It should be noted that the unit is unable to detect drop-offs at a depth less than 4 or 5 inches, and cannot signal an alarm when approaching a step from a distance of less than 45 inches.

Mobility curriculum adaptations
After the orientation and mobility evaluation has been performed, the appropriate orthopedic device(s) prescribed, and

physical therapy (e.g., gait training) completed, instruction can begin. The format for teaching indoor mobility skills to the physically handicapped blind is not radically different from the standard orientation and mobility training sequence. In developing program adaptations, one needs to consider the person's physical limitations as well as the type of device he or she is using.

Since the goal of any mobility training program is to maximize independence within the limits of the client's capabilities, the instructor must guard against limiting expectations. Flexibility, creativity, and some trial and error must be part of any program.

In some cases, a person may need to depend on a guide a great deal of the time. Instruction with this individual should stress using the guide as a tool for independence, not as someone to do all the work. The client should be responsible for his or her own decision making. In order to make decisions, the client should become knowledgeable in accessibility requirements for his or her own needs, soliciting aid by phone, planning routes, and wheelchair maintenance.

Based on our experience in teaching mobility to a number of physically handicapped blind clients, we have compiled adaptive methods of teaching selected indoor travel skills to people using walkers and wheelchairs. The techniques shown in Box 1 are basic in nature and are not meant to be an exhaustive listing. They are presented to give instructors a starting point for creative problem solving to meet the needs of their multiply handicapped clients.

References

Farmer, L. (1980). Mobility devices. In R. Welsh & B. Blasch (eds.), *Foundations of orientation and mobility*. New York: American Foundation for the Blind.

Morrissette, D.L., Goodrich, G.L., & Hennessey, J.J. (1981). A followup study of the Mowat Sensor's applications, frequency of use and the maintenance reliability. *Journal of Visual Impairment & Blindness,* **75**, 244-247.

Weinstock, R. (1982). Resources on mobility for the physically handicapped. *Journal of Visual Impairment & Blindness,* **76**, 317-318.

Cathy L. Coleman, orientation and mobility specialist; Robin F. Weinstock, M.Ed., supervisor of mobility training, Nevil Institute for Rehabilitation & Service, 919 Walnut St., Philadelphia, PA 19107.

Orientation and Mobility for the Low Functioning Deaf-Blind Child

D.R. Geruschat

Abstract: Describes how to do an initial evaluation, establish rapport, set realistic goals, and establish a training program. Stresses that a team approach is vital.

"Where do I start?" This is a common question that exemplifies the fear and frustration mobility instructors experience when confronted with the low functioning student. Our university training, internship experiences, and most of the employment opportunities focus on the development of orientation skills, cane techniques, and the use of low vision devices to help clients achieve their employment goals or maintain an independent living situation. Most clients are adventitiously blinded adults, with visual impairment as their primary, or only, disability. When beginning to work with the low functioning deaf-blind population, we experience a drastic change of our program goals. Now the development of sensory skills, spatial concepts, and simple route travel become integral parts of our teaching. If we are to succeed with this population, we must modify our teaching approaches as well as our goals.

The following program was developed over two years of work at the Upsal Day School for Multi-Handicapped Blind Children in Philadelphia, Pennsylvania. I have provided a general overview of orientation and mobility services with in-depth descriptions of the evaluative and program-planning processes. Many areas of our program were developed in conjunction with other specialists, and will be briefly mentioned in the hope that you will seek out the expertise of these specialists, as they are the ones to whom you must eventually turn; you cannot teach mobility in isolation. If your goal is a successful program, you must work with those involved with your student.

What is low functioning?
Before we begin this overview, I feel it is important to discuss the term *low func-*

Based on a paper given at the Wisconsin Workshop: Services for Deaf-Blind Persons, Madison, Wisconsin, April 30 and May 1, 1979.

tioning. I have been to many schools and workshops where the descriptor low functioning was used for a wide range of abilities. More often than not, I felt that my experiences with, and criteria of, low functioning students were different from those of other professionals in the field. Although I have no specific cut-off for low functioning, there are a few guidelines that help to keep this term in perspective.

First is the long-range goal for the student. Students who are not being prepared for a sheltered workshop because of the severity of their disability can generally be thought of as low functioning. The long-range goal for this type of student is most often acquisition of daily living skills. The second criterion is type of living situation anticipated. Institutionalization or some type of constant-care group home generally indicates a low functioning individual. While this is not a definitive analysis of what constitutes a low functioning individual, it gives us a common understanding of the type of students I am talking about.

Initial evaluation
The most important activity when beginning services for this population is doing a thorough evaluation. Figure 1 shows the mobility evaluation form which our staff developed. For each area, I have provided a sample list of questions which may give an insight into the kinds of information we generally looked for. Keep in mind that this is used only as a guide. For each student, you will expand and change the evaluation to obtain a complete picture of your new student's daily function. For this reason, we leave space to write comments after each item. Many answers require written descriptions of responses to accurately document your observations.

Visual evaluation
This category is described by Jose, Smith, and Shane (1980). It is the same evaluation that the mobility staff used.

Medications and restrictions
This is an area many people overlook. Often, knowing the type of medication a child takes can give you a clue as to why he or she is acting in a certain way or responding in a certain way. It is important to know time of day and effects of the drug. If the drug is taken at one o'clock and the effects are reduction of equilibrium, blurry vision, and sleepiness, you would probably want to schedule your mobility lesson before one o'clock or late in the day, when the effects of the drug are not impairing the child's ability to learn.

Other specialists
Everyone who works with the child is a valuable resource of information for understanding the whole child, and you should become familiar with their program of instruction. It may be that the most important consultants are the parents. Are your findings consistent with the parents' experiences in the home? Since your student spends most of his or her time at home, this valuable information resource should not be overlooked.

Mode of communication
This includes the child's method of communicating with the teacher and the teacher's method of communicating with the child. Does the child use signs or is the child verbal? What signs or words does the child know? Some very low functioning students may communicate through a behavioral response.

Body awareness/ environmental awareness
This is a very general category that can be approached in a number of ways. Sensory awareness and interactions with classroom staff and peers are the initial categories we emphasized. Important information includes whether or not the child recognizes familiar objects or caregiver and how the child receives and processes information. In later assessment procedures, more traditional tests of concept development and body image were used.

Description of child's movement
Does the student crawl, walk, etc.? What are the student's posture and gait? Are orthoptics, such as Canadian crutches or leg braces, needed? Also included are the types of protective techniques, obstacle avoidance, and balance problems.

Behavior management
This is a very important area to understand if you want to work successfully with these children. Does the child have a specific behavior modification program?

Classroom #: _____

Child's name: _____ Date of birth: _____

Cause of visual difficulty: _____

Onset: _____

Secondary visual conditions: _____

Visual evaluation: O.D. _____ O.S. _____

Fields: _____

Additional comments: _____

Other disabilities: _____

Which is the primary disability? _____

Medications/restrictions: _____

Other specialists: _____

Mode of communication: Singing, verbal, etc. _____

Receptive abilities: Does the child react to auditory command from teacher? _____

Expressive abilities: Signs or words child knows _____

Body awareness/environmental awareness: _____

Does child recognize familiar objects or caregiver? _____

What kind of interaction does child have with the staff? _____

What kind of interaction does child have with his/her peers? _____

How does the child receive and process information? _____

Description of child's movement: Is the child ambulatory? _____

Are there any postural or gait abnormalities? _____

Are orthoptics involved? If yes, how and what kind? _____

Does the child have protective reflexes? _____

Does the child have a balance problem? _____

Behavior management: Does the child have a specific behavior modification program? What behaviors are reinforced? How? What behaviors are being extinguished? How?

_____

What is the child's reinforcer? _____

Additional comments: Is the child toilet trained? _____

What are the warning signs? _____

Figure 1. Mobility evaluation.

What behaviors are being reinforced or extinguished? What is the child's reinforcer? Each child is handled in a different manner, so you must be flexible enough to work with other team members to develop a consistent approach to managing a student's behavior.

Additional comments
This category is for the multitude of questions that are generated by observing the student.

If you have never worked with this population before, you may find yourself rushing through an evaluation and settling into teaching the one area in which you feel most secure. Don't do it! The best way to avoid this pitfall is to learn how to do a thorough evaluation—and do one. This is the key to successful instruction. Ultimately, it will save time, guide you in setting priorities, and set the tone for a positive relationship with your new student.

Establishing rapport
When personal contact with the student occurs, begin in the classroom. Keep the environment and activity the same. If the student is having individual instruction from the teacher, assume the teacher's role. If the activity is a class activity, sit next to the child and begin with casual interaction. In this way, only one variable is presented at a time. Continue this approach in your own personal and creative way until you and your new student feel

comfortable together. At this point, I would take the student out of the classroom setting. Now the environment is the new variable. Use the same activities as in the classroom but change the room. Finally, expand your activities. Take a walk, play a game, anything which develops a positive, pleasant interaction.

Daily routine
As your relationship develops, certain activities will evolve into a time and type routine. Some children are very sensitive to any change of schedule, so it may be necessary not only to have your lessons at the same time of day, but also to introduce your activities in the same order. This is useful for helping the student to feel comfortable and secure with you. You will find that these children function best when they can anticipate activities. As your students expect activities, you will be able to expect and require consistent levels of performance. At this point, you and your student should know each other and feel comfortable together. As interaction with your student progresses, try to answer four very important questions: 1) What is the preferred avenue for taking in information? 2) How do the senses interact to process information? 3) Where is the best learning space? and 4) How long is the attention span? I do not include these questions in the initial evaluation because the answers may vary as the environment, instructor, and activities change.

Date ____________

Terminal objective: ____

____

____

Criterion: ____

☐ Initial evaluation ☐ Weekly follow-up

P- Physical cue V- Verbal Cue A- Auditory Cue I- Independent

Landmark	*Technique*	*Orientation*
Front door Step down	Square off Head up Shoulders back	 Reach out with right hand to find windows of foyer
Outside foyer	Trailing	Right hand
Stone wall	Trailing	Right hand
Corner of building	Trailing	Turn right
Downspout	Square off	Turn left Back to wall
Pillar	Line of direction	Place pillar on right side
Step down	Head up Shoulders back	Stop!

Figure 2. Form for analyzing and planning a route.

Relevant and realistic goals
Now that the child has been evaluated, we turn our attention to setting goals. These students have many needs which we could plan for. So how do we decide which goals to work on first? In deciding which goals are relevant, keep in mind Webster's definition: relevant means *applicable.* Does the acquisition of a skill apply in the context of his/her environment? Is it functional? Keep in mind that skill acquisition is not our goal. The functional application of that skill is.

Three program areas
In program planning, I generally divide the lesson into three major areas. The first area is sensory stimulation. Activation of the senses and striving toward optimal use of all the senses is a never-ending process which is worked on daily. Through consultation with the teacher, vision specialist, auditory specialist, physical therapist, and occupational therapist, many possibilities for a sensory stimulation program can be generated. Some of these people may already have a sensory stimulation program which you can incorporate into your daily routine.

The second major area is concept development. With very low functioning students, this generally means body awareness. Activities should include multisensory cues that require manipulation of specific body parts. For example, we could use a vibrator to tactually stimulate our legs. Then we could play a tambourine on our legs for tactual or auditory cues. Finally, we could have the student shine a light on his or her legs. It is important to place your student in situations where all available senses are used to experience a particular concept. For students who need work on spatial concepts, I found the method proposed by Hill (1971) to be a useful beginning. Lydon and McGraw (1973) is also a helpful resource. Since these sources were written with the higher functioning students in mind, it will be necessary to adapt these activities for each individual student. For example, in Lydon and McGraw (1973), their suggestions for auditory activities include bouncing a ball and having the student count the bounces, or following a sound in a straight line. To adapt these activities, we might see if the student can attend to the bouncing of a ball, or move toward the source of a sound. When adapting activities, be creative; present your material in an enjoyable way.

The final area is route travel. In selecting routes, always remember: Is it applicable? Does the student's independence increase once the route is learned? Commonly prescribed routes are to the bathroom, coatrack, cafeteria, dorm room, and front door. From the information obtained in your initial evaluation, and by discussing routes with the team members, you will be able to identify routes that are relevant to the student's daily routine.

Figure 2 shows a form that may be helpful in analyzing and planning your route. It is essential that your route be well planned. If there are best ways to travel the route, examine the alternatives carefully. Make your decision based on your evaluation of the student's abilities and needs.

It is of the utmost importance that you discuss and plan goals with the interdisciplinary team. When you plan with a team, you are better able to work with the whole child. You work together to solve the problems each student presents. You cannot do it alone.

When planning, three points should be remembered: 1) this is a team approach; 2) you need a well-thought-out and documented plan to work from; and 3) this plan can and should be changed as additional information about the child is learned.

Collecting data to show progress

This is where proper lesson planning is a must. We know that the learning process is slow and at times it seems nonexistent. However, documenting the daily activities will often graphically demonstrate progress. The team members can give you assistance in setting up charts and graphs for data collection. Professionals who have worked with your student in the past know how sensitive your system should be and can supply you with answers to most of your questions. If a behavioral psychologist is on staff, I suggest that you use this person's expertise in establishing the appropriate documentation.

Conclusion

Orientation and mobility services for the low functioning deaf-blind student are at an infantile stage. The literature, university training programs, and internship placements do not provide an extensive body of knowledge or experiences. As I stressed throughout my paper, the knowledge is gained by working within a team, not outside of the team. Combine your knowledge of orientation and mobility with the knowledge and experiences of other professions. By working with other professionals, you will gain the perspective which is necessary for establishing realistic goals and adapting methodologies.

Teaching the low functioning student can be one of the most challenging and rewarding experiences in your career. It demands creativity, hard work, and willingness to explore uncharted waters.

Finally, the emphasis when answering the question, "Where do I start?" is not on the word *where*; the emphasis should be on the word *start*. Get out there, learn by doing. The answers are not in a book, a university course, or a conference. We all must work hard and find the answers through our experiences.

References

Hill, E.W. (1970; 1971). The formation of concepts involved in body position in space. *Education of the Visually Handicapped*, **2**, 112-115; **3**, 21-25.

Lydon, W.T. & McGraw, M.L. (1973). *Concept development of visually handicapped children*. New York: American Foundation for the Blind.

Duane R. Geruschat, orientation and mobility specialist, Center for the Blind, Philadelphia, Pennsylvania.

Orientation and Mobility for the Blind Multiply Handicapped Young Child

R.K. Harley; R.G. Long; J.B. Merbler; T.A. Wood

Abstract: The purpose of this study was to develop and validate a programmed instructional program in orientation and mobility for blind multiply handicapped infants and toddlers below the developmental age of 3 years. Scales were developed for each of four major areas: motor development, cognitive development, movement and touch, and sound localization. Programmed instruction training materials were developed for each of these scales. The scales and programmed instruction were then field-tested with 22 multiply handicapped blind infants and toddlers functioning between 0 and 3 years of age. The children who received intervention from trainers using the programmed instructional materials demonstrated significant performance gains over the control subjects in the areas of cognitive development and movement and touch.

An important trend in the provision of orientation and mobility (O&M) services for visually impaired individuals is the extension of these services to young multiply impaired blind children. Since parents, preschool teachers, or nurse's aides provide most of the caregiving for these children in their early years, it seems important to provide instruction in the development of basic skills which would enable them to move about more efficiently in their homes.

An effective intervention program is always based on a careful assessment of the child's abilities. Bourgeault, Harley, DuBose, and Langley (1977) described an assessment procedure for multiply handicapped visually impaired children which resulted in a prescriptive program in the areas of motor, language, cognitive-adaptive, and social self-care skills. Mori and Olive (1978) made suggestions for an infancy intervention program in gross motor, sensory, cognitive, and fine motor skills. Felix and Spungin (1978), in a national survey of preschool services for the visually impaired, noted that training included visual efficiency, visual motor, body awareness, spatial orientation,

socialization, self-concept, auditory discrimination, self-help skills, and cognitive development. Recent research by Merbler and Wood (1984) suggests that very fundamental motor, sensory, and cognitive concepts normally acquired during the first 2 to 3 years of life are significantly related to later mobility performance.

Although programs have been reported in the literature regarding orientation and mobility for multiply handicapped blind preschool children (Moore, 1970), very little research can be found concerning the most effective methods of teaching these skills. Fraiberg (1977) noted that a prolonged period of immobility existed during the first year of life of the young blind child. It was not until late in the first year of development that the child reached for an object on sound cue alone. This resulting immobility posed a serious problem by limiting the ability to explore and discover objects in the environment. Bower (1982) concluded that the blind infant is unresponsive to most auditory stimuli because of inability to control the auditory stimulation that is delivered to it by others. Adelson and Fraiberg (1976) noted that the prolonged period of immobility during the blind child's first year could be shortened by an intervention program based upon uniting sound and touch. This intervention program was emphasized in the child-parent relationship and later in the play experiences given to the child.

Harley, Wood, and Merbler (1980) investigated the use of programmed instructional procedures for training prerequisite and limited mobility skills in multiply impaired blind children aged 2 to 5 years developmentally. The results of that study indicated that severely multiply impaired children could benefit from systematic instruction in mobility. In a subsequent study, Harley and Merbler (1980) successfully applied these programmatic techniques to multiply impaired low vision children who were developmentally comparable to the children of their earlier project. Although these studies demonstrated that programmed instruction in orientation and mobility was feasible for multiply impaired blind and low vision children, they did not address the needs of the youngest potential recipients of mobility services—blind multiply handicapped infants and toddlers from birth to 3 years.

Purpose
The primary objective of this project was to develop and validate a programmed instructional program in orientation and mobility for blind multiply handicapped infants and toddlers below the developmental age of three. The manual to be developed was to consist of an assessment instrument and programmed instruction for use by parents, teachers, and paraprofessionals. The assessment instrument was to be designed to evaluate children's developmental levels in the areas of motor, cognitive, and sensory skills. The programmed instruction was to be designed so that purpose, activity goal setting, materials, and the activity description were provided for each item on the scale. Each lesson was to be programmed in small, sequential steps with directions to the trainer showing how to start the activity, what to say, what to do, and when to proceed to the next step in the program.

Method
Subjects
A total of 25 multiply handicapped children, geographically located in three states, met the selection criteria for participation in the study. The criteria included:
• range in chronological age from birth to 7 years, 2 months;
• visual acuity of light perception or less, as documented by inability to visually fixate on or track a penlight held 8 inches from the child's face at eye level;
• posess at least one additional handicapping condition; and

Full support for this research was provided by U.S. Department of Education Grant #G008400665. The authors wish to thank Beth Langley for her part in developing the materials for this study.

• function on a preschool level below 3 years, 4 months, as determined by the Bayley Scales of Infant Development.

Three of the 25 children did not complete the study because of health problems and relocation. Demographic data indicated that the mean chronological age (CA) for the 22 children was 3 years, 2.5 months, with a range from 3 months to 7 years, 2 months. The developmental ages for the children ranged from 1 month to 3 years, 4 months, with a mean developmental age of 7.59 months. A total of 13 males and 9 female subjects comprised the experimental and control groups. Thirteen of the subjects resided in Alabama, five were in Indiana, and four were in Tennessee. Thirteen of the children were trained at home and the others were taught in preschool programs.

Materials
The first step in developing the scales for the subjects was to define the domains and the scales item content. Based on the review of literature and recommendations from early childhood educators and O&M specialists, three major curricular areas were selected to be addressed in the materials. The areas of cognitive, motor, and sensory development were selected because they seemed to be most important for the development of independent movement in young visually impaired children. Sensory development was divided into the two components of sound localization and movement and touch.

By further examination of the research literature and existing developmental scales for infants and young children, key skills appropriate to visually impaired children were selected. These skills were adapted for visually impaired children and reviewed by the consultants and advisory committee for the project. The items on the adapted scales were tried with selected visually impaired children functioning between 0 and 2 years of age. Nineteen items for cognitive, 15 items for motor, 15 items for movement and touch, and 10 items for sound localization were finally included in the assessment format for the scale (Figure 1). Each behavior was specified in the criterion-referenced assessment scale, along with the materials needed to assess the behavior, the procedure for conducting the assessment, the criterion for scoring the observed behavior, and the scoring procedure.

The format for the scale was designed to adhere to four guidelines. The first guideline was that the scale would follow

Figure 1. Behaviors included in the mobility scales.

I. Motor scale

1. Rolls from side to back.
2. Rolls from back to side.
3. Rolls from stomach to back.
4. Rolls from back to stomach.
5. Rolls from back to sitting position.
6. Rolls from stomach to sitting.
7. Rolls from supported sitting to stomach.
8. Rolls from supported sitting to back.
9. Maintains sitting posture.
10. Moves from stomach to hands and knees.
11. Creeps forward on hands and knees.
12. Moves from hands and knees to kneeling.
13. Moves from hands and knees to sitting.
14. Moves to standing from kneeling.
15. Maintains balance in standing and turning to reach for an object.

II. Sensory scale: Movement and touch

1. Reacts to and tolerates touch.
2. Reacts to and tolerates movement.
3. Holds object in hand.
4. Seeks out object after it touches child.
5. Reaches toward toy.
6. Reaches for and grasps toy.
7. Localizes point of touch on body.
8. Pats and/or tactually explores objects.
9. Explores container.
10. Fingers hole in pegboard.
11. Places block in formboard.
12. Locates last hole and inserts peg.
13. Places circle and square in formboard.
14. Places blocks in reversed formboard.
15. Distinguishes two indoor surfaces.

III. Sensory scale: Awareness and localization of sound

1. Reacts to sound.
2. Makes a grasping motion in response to sound.
3. Turns toward sound.
4. Reaches hand towards a soundmaking toy after grasping the toy.
5. Reaches toward a soundmaking toy after touching the toy.
6. Reaches hand toward soundmaking toy after hearing the toy.
7. Reaches hand toward soundmaking toy placed directly in front of the child.
8. Grasps soundmaking toy placed in front or to either side of the child.
9. Moves toward source sound.
10. Moves toward, locates, and grasps sound source.

IV. Cognition

1. Orients to two sounds.
2. Takes hand or toy to mouth.
3. Searches for object when removed from grasp.
4. Swipes at or hits suspended toy.
5. Holds one object in each hand.
6. Pats or feels object contacted.
7. Searches for dropped object.
8. Reaches around barrier to get toy.
9. Drops one object to obtain third.
10. Removes toy from small box with lid.
11. Recognizes the reversal of an object.
12. Places one block in container.
13. Demonstrates functional use of objects.
14. Pulls string horizontally to secure toy.
15. Matches three pairs of common objects (2 cups, 2 shoes, 2 dolls).
16. Places 6-8 blocks in container.
17. Removes small object from narrow-necked bottle.
18. Identifies three common objects.
19. Points to basic body parts.

a criterion-referenced format based on items which were arranged in a sequence similar to that followed by normally developing young children. The second guideline was that the scale would follow a criterion-referenced format based on direct observation of the behaviors of interest. The third guideline was that the scale could be administered with minimal verbal interaction between the examiner and child.

The fourth guideline was that the instruments could be administered easily by teachers or parents. The administration procedures were carefully described for each item, including positions of the examiner and the child, the presentation procedure, the materials needed, the behavior to be observed, the criterion for scoring, and the scoring procedure.

In general assessment procedure, the examiner presented the task to the child, observed the child's response, rated the response, and scored the rating on the scale protocol. The administration time varied from about 60 to 90 minutes, depending largely on the attention span of the child.

Reliability
Interrater reliability was computed on 16 of the participants across three sites during the pretest phase of the project. The procedure for conducting interrater reliability involved one experienced clinician administering all the assessment scales to each of the 16 children, while two raters observed and scored assessment protocols independent of one another. Percent agreement of two raters for all scale items averaged 90.6 percent. On the posttest, test-retest reliability data were obtained for the same 16 children. One clinician administered the posttest assessment to a child, and then readministered the test within five days. Percent agreement on all scale items averaged 94.5 percent using this method (Tawney & Gast, 1984).

Validity
In order to achieve some degree of validity, the initial items for the four scales were selected from observations of the authors and others (Fraiberg, 1977; Bower, 1982) who had worked with visually impaired young children. A comprehensive review of various infant and preschool scales used with non-visually impaired children was also used in the development of the scales. The items were revised after trying out the items with visually impaired infants and toddlers. Finally, the items were reviewed by nine consultants who had considerable experience in working with visually impaired young children in the areas represented on these scales.

Development of the programmed instruction
The programmed instruction for the project was organized into the same four separate components as the scale: cognitive, motor, movement and touch, and sound localization. Each scale item was matched by a corresponding item in the programmed instruction. The tasks in the program were sequenced developmentally so that the child could progress from entry point to the terminal objective through successive approximations. The entire program was based on behavior modification procedures, using positive reinforcement as the child successfully achieved each pinpointed approximation of the step. Each lesson was divided according to activity goal, setting, materials, and suggested educational procedure. The educational procedure was divided according to "trainer does," "trainer says," and "child does." Each task in the program was divided into three levels. In Level A, the trainer physically guided the child through the entire task. In Level B, the trainer provided the child with some assistance by physically prompting the child through the beginning movements of the activity. In Level C, the trainer provided a cue, such as a tap, as a signal for the child to begin the movement required by the activity. In all levels, the child was given a verbal prompt in addition to the physical assistance. The overall goal of the training program was to enable the child to learn to perform successfully at the independent level (Level C) for six consecutive trials. Independent data sheets were provided for each activity so that the trainer could record data for the training trials.

Procedure
The wide geographical range of the study required the employment of a graduate assistant within each state. The graduate assistants were doctoral students enrolled at local universities at which each primary investigator was affiliated. Each graduate assistant was carefully trained and supervised in the use of assessment and intervention materials by the local investigator. The graduate assistants were primarily responsible for assessment, daily data collection, and home/center liaison.

Subjects were pretested, using the assessment scales of the instructional materials by the graduate assistants. Subjects' parents or teachers were encouraged to be present during the testing sessions. In some instances, it was necessary to schedule two testing sessions to insure a subject's cooperation. Individual prescriptive profiles were created for each subject based on the assessment results. Fourteen parents, four teachers, three nurse's aides, and one nurse provided the instruction.

Since only a very few children were identified who met the study's selection criteria, it was necessary to use an experimental design in which subjects served as both experimental and control conditions. Consequently, each subject was assigned intervention in at least one developmental area (e.g., Movement and Touch), and also simultaneously served as a control in at least one developmental area. The resulting design had elements of the "equivalent materials design" described by Campbell and Stanley (1963), and multitreatment design used by Atkinson (1968). Through this design, each subject was represented in each of the four developmental areas. However, a subject's status in a particular area could be either experimental or control. For example, a subject might be designated as experimental for the Cognitive, Motor, and Movement and Touch areas, and control status for the remaining area. Consequently, a total of 88 blocks or units of data were generated. Forty-five of these blocks were experimental, and 43 were control. Each developmental area had a total of 22 units. In each area, 11 units were experimental and 11 were control, with the exception of the Cognitive area, in which 12 units were experimental and 10 units were control. The decision regarding which areas would be experimental and which control for any particular subject was based on (1) a subject's relative need for intervention as indicated by the assessment profile (i.e., consistent with the manner in which the instrument would actually be used in an intervention setting), and (2) a general attempt to maintain equivalent numbers of experimental and control conditions within each intervention area. Although this approach to subject assignment would seem to lead to regression toward the mean confounding (Campbell & Stanley, 1963), the differences between subtest scores within subjects were not extreme. Furthermore, the use of this more prescriptive assignment method was thought to be more faithful to the actual use of the materials by teachers or parents.

Intervention was scheduled for 16 weeks. Those subjects enrolled in center-based programs received intervention through their regular teacher. Home-based subjects received intervention through their parents. During the 16-week intervention period, the intervention agents completed weekly progress reports that were returned to the graduate assistants. These progress reports were used for decision-making regarding advancement through the steps of the particular sessions. The graduate assistants usually visited the intervention sites biweekly.

Following the intervention period, each subject was posttested across all developmental areas, using the same assessment used for the pretest. In addition, the intervention agents completed a final evaluation of the material as a basis for revisions.

Results

Pre-posttest gain scores for the experimental and control conditions were used for all statistical analyses (Cook & Campbell, 1979). Gain scores were used as the dependent variable because of:

- non-equivalence of experimental and control condition pretest means, and
- the within-subject treatment design of the study.

Analysis of gain scores focuses on differences in the mean change between treatment conditions as opposed to differences in posttest means.

Table 1 presents several descriptive statistics computed on the data. Examination of Table 1 indicates both a higher mean gain and standard deviation for the experimental conditions in both the Home and Center settings. Pearson Product Moment Correlation Coefficients were computed between number of trials and gain scores to determine whether a relationship existed between trials and gain. This analysis was necessitated by the wide range in the number of training trials across subjects, as indicated by the high standard deviation for trials. The resulting coefficients of $r = .052$ (Experimental) and $4 = -.111$ (Control) were not significant.

A single factor (Treatment) repeated measures analysis of variance was used to analyze the overall effect of the training program. The difference between mean gains of subjects' experimental and control conditions was significant ($F(1,21) = 12.56$, $p < .002$), as noted in Table 2. The statistical validity of ANOVA techniques when applied to designs in which subjects were within both experimental and control conditions has been established in the literature (e.g., Shine, 1973).

A two-factor analysis of variance with one between (Setting) and one repeated (Treatment) factor was used to analyze the effect of training implemented in home- versus center-based settings. The primary comparison of interest, Setting, approached significance ($F(1,20) = 4.096$, $p < .054$). The Setting X Treatment interaction was not significant. The Treatment factor was significant ($F(1,20) = 10.93$, $p < .003$), as noted in Table 3.

A series of "t" tests was conducted to analyze subject gains within each skill area. Only two areas, Cognitive ($t(22) = 2.96$, $p < .007$) and Movement and Touch ($t(20) = 2.84$, $p < .009$) showed significant gain. The resulting "t" statistics for Motor ($t(20) = .418$) and Sound Localization ($t(20) = 1.309$) were not significant.

Results of the final written evaluations submitted by the intervention agents were largely formative, suggesting specific lessons that could be improved or were unclear. Overall, the parents and teachers who participated in the study were very pleased by the materials and the outcomes of their intervention efforts.

Discussion

The results of the statistical analyses suggest that the programmed intervention was generally successful, with statistically significant gains achieved in the Cognitive and Movement and Touch skill areas. The failure to obtain statistically significant gains in the Motor and Sound Localization areas can probably be attributed to the history of the subjects during the study. Several children were concurrently receiving physical therapy and/or classroom activities which were similar to the intervention program. Consequently, the control conditions for Motor and Sound Localization were at high risk of confounding.

In contrast, the Cognitive and Movement and Touch activities were relatively unique to the intervention program, and far fewer control condition gains were observed in these areas. The general stability of the control conditions during the study suggests that the treatments were relatively orthogonal. This observation is important since a repeated treatment design of the type employed in this study can be confounded by non-independent treatment conditions (i.e., intervention in one area directly affects performance in another, non-intervened-upon behavior).

It is impossible to determine whether intervention in one area contributed to improvement in a second intervention area in those instances where subjects were placed in two experimental conditions. However, the various combinations of treatments (e.g., intervention on Motor and Cognitive, control on Sensory, versus intervention on Motor and Sensory, control on Cognitive) minimized this possibility.

The outcomes of the analysis of home versus center program implementation suggests that parents can effectively execute an intervention program in the area of pre-mobility for their children. However, the high variability of gain scores within the home condition suggests that some parents may have been more successful than others. The large difference between the mean gain scores of the home trainees (20.85) and center trainees (8.00) should not be construed as a marked superiority of home-based training. First, the difference was not statistically significant. Second, the training which occured in the home setting was very specific and intensive regarding the intervention areas. Center-based training

Table 1. Selected descriptive statistics for the study.

Setting	Condition	Posttest mean gain	SD	Mean trials	Trials SD
Home	Experimental	21.46	18.99	1,032.69	1,040.11
Home	Control	8.69	11.47		
Center	Experimental	8.00	6.60	906.11	496.13
Center	Control	3.11	3.11		

Table 2. Analysis of variance summary for treatment effects.

Source	Sum of squares	Degrees of freedom	Mean square	F
Blocks/subjects	5,672.55	21		
treatment	855.36	1	855.36	12.56*
error	1,430.64	21	68.13	

*$p < .002$

Table 3. Analysis of variance summary for setting.

Source	Sum of squares	Degrees of freedom	Mean square	F
Between blocks/ subjects				
setting	964.26	1	964.26	4.10*
error	4,708.29	20	235.42	
Within blocks/ subjects				
treatment	717.58	1	717.58	10.93**
setting/treatment	117.58	1	117.58	1.79
error	1,313.06	20	65.65	

*$p < .054$
**$p < .003$

included additional areas of instruction which could make the training effect broader (i.e., lower gains in more areas in contrast to higher gains in very restricted areas). This conclusion is somewhat supported by the mean trial data which indicated that more trials occurred in the home setting (X = 1,032.69) compared to the center setting (S = 906.11).

The outcomes of this study suggest that multiply handicapped blind infants and toddlers can benefit from carefully programmed instruction. Further, it seems that this training can be effectively provided by either a teacher or the child's parents. This finding should be particularly encouraging for those parents who do not have easy access to a center-based intervention program. Although the findings reported in this study are statistically significant, they must nonetheless be interpreted with a degree of caution. The relatively small number of subjects in conjunction with the essentially quasi-experimental design (Cook & Campbell, 1979) necessitated by the field settings could limit the ability to generalize the findings. Although no pattern of results in the data suggested confounding, replication of the study with a larger group of subjects and a more traditional control group would enhance the reliability of the findings.

The recommendations of the intervention agents were used to revise the instructional lessons. This modified version of the materials was critiqued by a group of field consultants who are recognized experts in the area of developmental intervention for visually impaired multiply handicapped young children. The suggestions of these reviewers have been incorporated into a final revision of the materials which is under contract for publication. Overall, the modified version was deemed by the field consultants to be valid, and they supported its potential usefulness with blind multiply handicapped infants and toddlers.

References

Adelson, E. & Fraiberg, S. (1976). Sensory deficit and motor development in infants blind from birth. In *The effects of and other impairments on early development* (Jastrzembska, X.S., Ed.). New York: American Foundation for the Blind.

Atkinson, R.C. (1968). Computerized instruction and learning process. *American Psychologist,* **23**, 225-239.

Bourgeault, S.F., Harley, R.K., DuBose, R.F., & Langley, M.B. (1977). Assessment and programming for blind children with severely handicapping conditions. *Journal of Visual Impairment & Blindness,* **71**, 49-53.

Bower, T.G.R. (1982). *Development in infancy.* San Francisco: W.H. Freeman.

Campbell, D.T. & Stanley, J.C. (1963). *Experimental and quasi-experimental designs for research.* Chicago: Rand McNally.

Cook, T.D. & Campbell, D.T. (1979). *Quasi-experimentation: Design and analysis issues for field settings.* Chicago: Rand McNally.

Felix, L.F. & Spungin, S.J. (1978). Preschool services for the visually handicapped: A national survey. *Journal of Visual Impairment & Blindness,* **73**, 59-66.

Fraiberg, S.H. (1977). *Insights from the Blind.* New York: Basic Books.

Harley, R.K. & Merbler, J.B. (1980). Development of an orientation and mobility program for multiply impaired low vision children. *Journal of Visual Impairment & Blindness,* **74**(1), 9-14.

Harley, R.K., Wood, T.A. & Merbler, J.B. (1980). An orientation and mobility program for multiply impaired blind children. *Exceptional Children,* **46**(5), 326-331.

Merbler, J.B. & Wood, T.A. (1984). Predicting orientation and mobility proficiency in mentally retarded visually impaired children. *Education and Training of the Mentally Retarded,* **19**(3), 228-230.

Moore, M.E. (1970). *Developing body image and skills of orientation, mobility and social competence in preschool, multiply handicapped blind children.* Doctoral dissertation, University of Pittsburgh. Ann Arbor, MI: University Microfilms, No. 70-20.

Mori, A.G. & Olive, J.E. (1978). The blind and visually handicapped mentally retarded: Suggestions for intervention in infancy. *Journal of Visual Impairment & Blindness,* **72**, 273-279.

Shine, L.L. (1973). A multi-way analysis of variance for single-subject design. *Educational and Psychological Measurement,* **33**, 633-636.

Tawney, J.W. & Gast, D.L. (1984). *Single subject research in special education.* Columbus, OH: Charles E. Merrill.

Randall K. Harley, Ph.D., professor, Dept. of Special Education, Peabody College for Teachers of Vanderbilt University, Nashville, TN; Richard G. Long, Ph.D., research health scientist, Research and Demonstration Center, Veterans Administration, Decatur, GA; John B. Merbler, Ph.D., professor, Dept. of Special Education, Ball State University, Muncie, IN; Thomas A. Wood, Ed.D., associate professor, Dept. of Special Education and Rehabilitation, Auburn University, Auburn, AL.

Orientation and Mobility for Severely and Profoundly Retarded Blind Persons

M.M. Uslan

Abstract: The lack of attention to orientation and mobility for both severely and profoundly retarded blind persons is seen as an interdisciplinary problem that educators for the retarded and educators for the blind—especially mobility instructors—can and should remediate. The scant literature that does exist is reviewed and suggestions are made for improving locomotor skills, organizing physical exercises, teaching orientation skills, and teaching cane travel.

In a timely article documenting the growth of programs for blind mentally retarded children, Maurice I. Tretakoff (1977) highlighted an important fact: Educators of the blind and educators of the retarded need each other if the growth and benefits of their services are to be sustained. Professional interdependence is particularly important in programs for blind persons who are either severely or profoundly retarded. Educators of the retarded who deal with problems posed by blindness may find themselves ill-equipped, without professional help, to meet all the perplexities of orientation and mobility. The mobility practitioner may also, without help, be inadequately versed in techniques of behavior modification. These facts need not be particularly distressing, since any establishment serving blind retarded persons—state hospital or training center, developmental center, special residential facility—should easily offset the particular shortcomings of each kind of training by allowing professionals to swap "tools." The exchange of practical and theoretical resources among professionals should not be considered a mere convenience; it is, in fact, essential, because literature treating mobility of blind persons who are either severely or profoundly retarded is scarce. The methods sketched here will, it is hoped, provoke educators of the retarded and educators of the blind—especially mobility practitioners—to devote more

attention to approaches to teaching orientation and mobility.

Assessment

A few appropriate analytical tools do exist for assessing the mobility potential of those who are either severely or profoundly retarded. Although not designed specifically for the blind, the AAMP Index (Webb, 1969) provides useful material for the mobility practitioner. Webb identified four areas of underdevelopment in the profoundly retarded: awareness, movement, manipulation of the environment, and posture and locomotion. In addition to a rating scale based on her symptomatology of profound retardation, Webb also outlined, in a logical format, techniques of sensory motor training. Her outline identified sense stimulated therapy activity, and equipment for each target behavior.

The Peabody Mobility Scale (Harley, Wood, & Merbler, 1976) is a unique orientation and mobility assessment instrument designed for a wide range of multiply handicapped blind children. The assessment areas are motor development, sensory skills, concept development, and orientation and mobility skills. It also includes a programmed instruction component in each of the assessment areas. For some lessons, prerequisite training activities are provided. Unfortunately, the authors found that nonverbal children function at a level too low to benefit from training activities. Nevertheless, the Peabody Mobility Scale is important as a methodically designed and carefully validated orientation and mobility assessment instrument for multiply handicapped blind children.

Locomotor skills

The institutionally ingrained habit of moving blind residents in "herds" may seem efficient to an attendant, but unfortunately this practice discourages residents' independent movement. Furthermore, when purposeful and controlled, independent movement can be more efficient than involuntary herding. All those in contact with residents when they are being moved can be involved in the institutional effort to encourage independent movement. For example, in-service training of attendants and aides might suggest alternatives to herding. Virtually every time aides must move residents, they can take advantage of the situation by encouraging the residents, one by one, to folllow.

Unless it is discouraged, the habit of tarrying also reduces the amount of satisfaction many retarded blind residents obtain in moving about. Severely and profoundly retarded residents troubled with extremely slow walking speed and short stridelength often do not respond to verbal and physical encouragement to "come," even when such urging is combined with receiving food as a reward. The slow-moving resident usually shifts his weight back on his heels with his trunk also shifted backward. An instructor's attempt to pull him forward only exaggerates this tendency since, in an effort to resist, the resident further increases the defensive reaction and the postural faults that accompany it (Figure 1).

An effective method of overcoming tarrying is to walk alongside the resident and apply gentle pressure from behind to encourage forward motion and promote a more normal walking speed. Miller (1969) has stated that head dominance is a feature in all normal movement and that the classic blind gait (weight shifted backward to the heels) is a defensive response to the lack of vision. By nudging from behind, the instructor can induce the reflex response to a loss of balance, forcing the resident to take a step forward. If the instructor continues with these gentle nudges, he can suppress the resident's defenses and facilitate the natural reflex. As in most instructional efforts with retarded persons, all those who come in contact with the individual should be actively engaged in the learning process by reinforcing correct technique.

Physical exercise

If it is important that severely and profoundly retarded children be encouraged

The author would like to thank Susan Stephens, a physical therapist and a graduate of the Boston College peripatology program, for her assistance in researching the problem of tarrying.

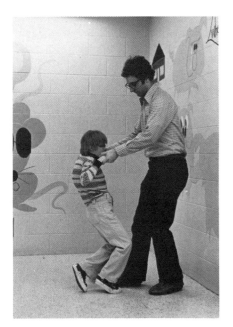
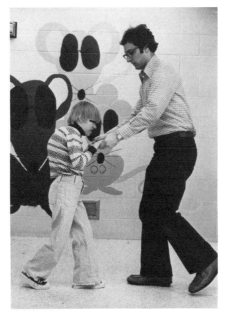

Figure 1. Since the slow-moving resident usually shifts his weight to the rear in walking, pulling him exaggerates the backward displacement of his weight and necessarily creates involuntary bodily resistance to the tow.

to exercise regularly, it is even more crucial that blind children, who are especially liable to the gross postural problems and listlessness caused by prolonged sitting around, be encouraged to move often. The pathological aspects of leisure make physical activity a matter of survival. Wilson (1974) has clearly described dayroom activity of the severely and profoundly retarded:

> This group of institutionalized patients simply deteriorated, the tendency being for most of them to sit in one place and indulge in strange mannerisms or produce inhuman sounds. There is no interaction, for most of them are non-verbal. At times they act aggressively toward one another in terms of their boredom and frustration. They have no model to copy. Interaction with staff comes only when there is a physical need to be met, or when they misbehave.

Again, all those who come in contact with the blind retarded resident must be involved in the effort to instruct (Figure 2).

Although the mobility practitioner is not a specialist in adaptive physical education, he can certainly be expected to organize rudimentary exercises to be done with apparatus and independent of it. Basic equipment should usefully augment a light calisthenic routine. A modest gym containing an exercise bicycle (the standard exercise bicycle is easily adapted for severely retarded blind residents), a horizontal ladder, a balance beam, a vestibular board,

exercise mats, and portable training stairs serve residents well and simply.

Orientation skills

Measuring social interaction and movement among 30 severely and profoundly retarded men, McGlinchey and Mitala (1975) found that residents were generally stationary. They spent virtually all of their time in one place in the dayroom;

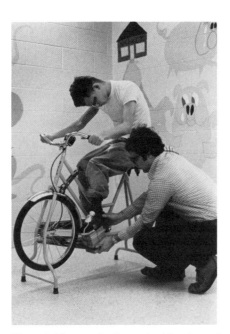
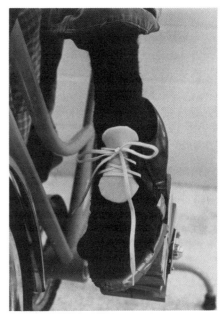

Figure 2. The standard exercise bicycle can be adapted for severely and profoundly retarded persons by building up the pedal height and by attaching an old pair of shoes to the built-up pedals.

their social interaction, including that which accompanied such obligatory staff assistance as toileting and feeding, was negligible. McGlinchey and Mitala attributed this unusually scant movement and social interaction to the residents' lack of ward orientation and total dependence on attendants. They contended that the residents' blindness hampered them more drastically than their profound retardation, because blindness seriously interfered with all aspects of the subjects' training to care for themselves.

To guide residents from one place to another, McGlinchey and Mitala affixed tactile cues to ward walls and implemented a training method which featured backward chaining. In backward chaining, the task is first broken down into discrete steps that can be thought of as links of a chain. Beginning from the destination, the resident is taught the final link first. Preceding links to the familiar parts of a chain are added until, finally, the starting position is taught. This system is sensibly uncomplicated and inexpensive.

More recently, Uslan (1976) has proposed a novel way of teaching ward design to direct residents by auditory clues. Uslan placed electronically triggered floor mats at critical turning points on a simple route from the dayroom to the dining room; when they stepped on these mats, residents activated strategically located speakers that played "food associated" music. This approach, intended to emphasize the intrinsic meaning of a clue or landmark, furnishes a good starting point for adding to and improving upon the simple system of McGlinchey and Mitala. It is, however, only applicable to residents who respond normally to auditory stimuli; it is rather elaborate and expensive and is relatively untested.

Use of the cane

Since cane travel demands a considerable degree of resourcefulness, teaching cane travel technique to retarded individuals has been traditionally limited to those who are only moderately retarded and have the intellectual and motor potential to travel independently to familiar destinations. For the more severely retarded, the cane can also be considered as a simple walking aid: it helps the person keep his balance, provides advance warning of danger, and samples the path of travel for changes in terrain. On the basis of Miller's (1976) analysis of the cane as a prosthetic device, one can legitimately describe the cane as an instinctive aid to locomotion. Thus, the cane might be considered as a device for improving the independent walking ability of blind individuals who are either severely or profoundly retarded.

When treated as a supervised outdoor activity, cane travel training can provide the retarded individual with a unique walking experience analogous to independent travel for the higher functioning blind. Additionally, cane travel training logically supplements the physical exercise program.

To learn basic diagonal technique or fundamental touch technique requires only that a resident can grip the cane and does not exhibit behavior problems likely to make use of the cane hazardous. Some residents who can grip the cane will begin to learn how to use it once an instructor has merely helped them to hold it and has tapped it in touch technique fashion, counting, "one-two, one-two" to establish a rhythm coordinated with walking. When they find it too difficult to master motor skills involved in the touch technique, residents may learn a simpler tapping technique in which the cane is held in the diagonal cross-body position. Having mastered at least a crude, basic technique that can be executed with relative independence, the resident is ready to embark on a straight line sidewalk route outside the ward.

It is difficult to see how the cane can be taught to blind persons who are either severely or profoundly retarded other than in a highly controlled leisure time setting. At Muscatatuck State Hospital and Training Center (a state institution for the retarded in Indiana), a relatively high functioning adult who was familiar with ward layout and the environment immediately outside the ward, was taught basic touch technique. After the resident had been given the cane for three weeks, the attendant staff (11 persons) were surveyed to determine what problems, if any, the cane introduced into the ward. The attendants considered the cane hazardous to the resident, other residents, and even employees. It was therefore recommended that the resident use the cane only when accompanied by an aide, attendant, or volunteer. Thus, cane travel must be considered as a supervised leisure time activity if it is to benefit the retarded individual.

At Muscatatuck State Hospital and Training Center, four severely retarded residents were also instructed in cane travel. The residents (20-25 years old) had acquired only minimal communication and self-help skills and their mobility skills were limited to ward travel necessary to fulfill basic needs. For them, the cane travel task was broken down into 11 steps:
1. Grasp cane.
2. Grasp cane at side of body.
3. Pivot wrist with cane in front of body.
4. Pivot wrist so that cane's arc approximates shoulder width.
5. Tap cane at shoulder width.
6. Tap cane at shoulder width while walking.
7. Distinguish grass from sidewalk with cane.
8. Walk between two sidewalk obstructions.
9. Turn around at obstructions.
10. Return to starting point.
11. Go to meaningful destinations with instructor.

After approximately one month of daily 45-minute lessons, the residents were evaluated. Figure 3 indicates that two of the four students achieved the objective of independent performance. Although less success was attained with the remaining two residents, it is clear that teaching cane travel to the blind who are either severely or profoundly retarded is worth the effort.

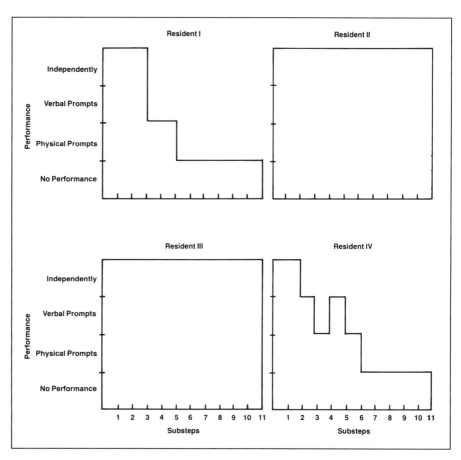

Figure 3. Mobility achievements of four severely retarded persons. Histograms show resident performance when taught 11 sub-steps of cane travel.

Solving the problems of movement and navigation experienced by the blind who are either severely or profoundly retarded often begins with the willingness to try out new ideas. Mobility practitioners at institutions for the retarded must relinquish conventional methods which are ill-designed to promote independent travel, and adopt only the simplest schemes to change residents' daily habits—schemes that reinforce more satisfying behavior and impart a sense of movement as a rewarding activity. Solutions to specific problems will arise over time, as increasing numbers of practitioners gain long experience in teaching orientation and mobility to blind persons who are either severely or profoundly retarded.

References

Harley, R.K., Wood, A., & Merbler, J.B. (1976). *The development of a program in orientation and mobility for multiply impaired blind children.* HEW Grant G007500596, George Peabody College for Teachers, Nashville, TN.

McGlinchey, M.A. & Mitala, R.F. (1975). Using environmental design to teach ward layout to severely and profoundly retarded blind persons: A proposal. *The New Outlook for the Blind, 69,* 168-171.

Miller, J. (1967). Vision, a component of locomotion. *Physiotherapy, 53,* 326-332.

Miller, J. (1969). The development or re-establishment of movement in patients with abnormal vision. *Australia Journal of Physiotherapy, 15*(4), 135-140.

Tretakoff, M.I. (1977). The evolution of programs for blind mentally retarded children in residential facilities. *Journal of Visual Impairment & Blindness, 71,* 29-33.

Uslan, M.M. (1976). Teaching basic ward layout to the severely retarded blind: An auditory approach. *The New Outlook for the Blind, 70,* 401-402.

Webb, R.C. (1969). Sensory motor training of the profoundly retarded. *American Journal of Mental Deficiency, 74,* 283-295.

Wilson, D.A. (1974). Teaching multiply handicapped blind persons in a state hospital. *The New Outlook for the Blind, 68,* 337-343.

Mark M. Uslan, lecturer, Boston College peripatology program.

OPPORTUNITIES

The critical question of what adult role
the visually impaired person with multiple
disabilities will fill is the focus of this section.
Solutions to the continuing gap between ability
and opportunity are suggested in these articles.

Employment of Deaf-Blind Rubella Students in a Subsidized Work Program

D.G. Busse; L.T. Romer; R.R. Fewell; P.F. Vadasy

Abstract: Recipients of training in a model vocational program for deaf-blind youth participated in a summer workshop placement. Three deaf-blind teenaged students were placed for four to eight weeks in a community-subsidized work program modeled on the Specialized Training Program. All students generalized assembly and self-help skills in which they had been trained, with peer tutor assistance, prior to placement. Their rates of productivity and supervisor contacts were similar to those of other work program employees. The results demonstrate the potential of individualized programming to meet the vocational needs of the adolescent deaf-blind rubella population in existing work programs for the severely handicapped.

The increase over the past decade in adult vocational programs for severely handicapped persons suggests possible opportunities for rubella deaf-blind youth who are approaching adulthood. This population, with sensory impairments that are often combined with intellectual and physical deficits as well as behavior problems, has rarely been considered as potential employees by sheltered-workshop staff.

However, with the development of successful subsidized work programs such as the Specialized Training Program (STP) (Bellamy, Horner, & Inman, 1979), in which severely retarded persons have begun to earn workshop wages far in excess of national sheltered-workshop norms (Bellamy, Borbeau, & Sowers, 1983), the possibility of subsidized employment as opposed to activity-center programming for the rubella population deserves serious consideration. The basic question that educators should ask regarding the educational needs of deaf-blind students has changed from "What activity-center program will best meet the needs of deaf-blind rubella persons?" to "What training at the high-school level can facilitate their movement into vocational programs?" This change is a significant one.

In the past, goals of educational programs for rubella youth involved moving the deaf-blind students slowly along the continuum of development demonstrated by normal children, regardless of the student's age. A more appropriate goal, particularly for those deaf-blind students of high-school age, is to provide specific training that prepares the students for a future that includes work and wages (Wilcox & Bellamy, 1982).

The model program

The Innovative Vocational Model for Deaf-Blind Youth Project at the University of Washington was a three-year federal contract seeking to develop a vocational training model for rubella deaf-blind youth of high-school age. The model was intended to reflect the actual job opportunities in the student's community. The basic classroom program that has been developed by this project involves the use of peer tutors who work one-on-one with assigned deaf-blind rubella high-school-age students for two hours each school day. One hour each day is devoted to vocational training, which consists of two or three different instructional programs. The second hour is devoted to practicing tasks previously learned under simulated work conditions. Tasks have varied, but are designed to simulate actual workshop jobs. One of the project's objectives was to provide supervised placement in a community setting for some of the project participants in the last year of the project.

The workshop survey

In 1981, project staff surveyed subsidized work programs in Washington state to determine which facilities viewed themselves as appropriate settings for placement of rubella deaf-blind students in the project who would soon turn 21. Efforts were directed at determining whether workshops already serving the severely retarded could also serve those rubella adults who were not only severely retarded, but also had multiple sensory impairments.

The initial survey revealed that very few workshops regarded themselves as appropriate settings for this population. Only 11 of 29 programs expressed any interest in working with project subjects or other deaf-blind individuals. Either rubella deaf-blind adults were considered to be clearly outside the specific disabled population served by the particular workshop, or the workshop staff felt that the additional skills and worker:staff ratios required for this population exceeded their resources. One particular group of subsidized work programs did, however, express interest in this population. These were facilities based upon the Specialized Training Program (STP) model developed at the University of Oregon. This model stresses limited program size (approximately 20 workers) and well-trained staff (four persons with proven skills in the area of behavioral management), and focuses upon serving only the severely retarded (Bellamy, Horner, & Inman, 1979). Discussions with STP staff led us to conclude that these particular programs had the greatest chance of success in working with rubella adults. These survey results were the basis for project efforts to develop a high-school vocational training program for rubella youth that would prepare them for their transition from school into subsidized employment in STP replication facilities.

Requirements for workshop placement

Once the transition into subsidized employment in STP replications or STP-like facilities was identified as an objective, the following questions had to be answered.

What skills should be taught to best facilitate the transition, and to what extent will these skills generalize to the new environment?

While ideally students should be taught tasks specific to the particular program in which they would eventually be placed, the difficulty of identifying exactly which programs would receive which trainees made such precise pretraining impossible. As we noted, not only did few programs identify themselves as potential sites for these students, but also the students would later require placements in their home communities, which were scattered all across the state. This meant these students were not residing in what would ultimately be their community setting upon graduation. In addition, even if a specific program were identified for each student, predicting accurately the exact work tasks that would be required in three or four years was very difficult. Consequently, we chose tasks that were either typical of STP programs (Romer, 1983) or that required similar generic skills (such as threading nuts, bagging items, or using a screwdriver).

Additionally, certain general skills or attributes were identified as being critical or necessary for successful transition into a subsidized program. These included the amount of training time required to learn new tasks; presence of self-stimulatory behaviors; self-care skills related to arrival at work, eating lunch, toileting, etc.; and ability to work with very little or no supervision for periods of up to one hour. Identification of these skills was accomplished through use of the workshop questionnaire developed by Mitaug, Hagmier, and Haring (1977).

What communication skills will subsidized program staff need in order to work with deaf-blind severely retarded workers?
An issue of great concern, if deaf-blind mentally retarded persons are to be integrated into general subsidized employment programs rather than segregated workshops developed specifically for them, is that of staff communication skills. Two conflicting philosophies exist. First, many workers with the deaf-blind had suggested to project staff that anyone working with a deaf-blind person should be a fluent signer, even if that deaf-blind person has only eight to ten receptive and virtually no expressive signs. The theory behind this demand is that the deaf-blind individual's constant exposure to sign language will facilitate sign language learning (Groht, 1958; Van Uden, 1970). On the other hand, analyses of the workplace reveal that very little communication actually occurs among the severely retarded in workshops, and therefore the low levels of communication between the deaf-blind severely retarded workers and staff are not cause for concern.

Also, workshop staff seldom possess signing skills unless the particular facility

serves deaf persons. The issue remains, then, as to whether workshop staff must receive extensive sign training prior to admitting deaf-blind workers, or whether training in a minimal number of signs (equivalent to the very limited vocabularies of most rubella persons) will suffice.

To what extent will self-stimulatory behaviors interfere with the deaf-blind worker's assimilation into the workshop setting, both in terms of decreased production and distraction of sighted handicapped workers?
The deaf-blind subjects in this project all exhibited self-stimulatory behaviors that tended to decrease production rates. The environmental survey we conducted revealed that staff in STP programs are familiar with the self-stimulatory behaviors of severely retarded persons. What we did not see during training, however, were dramatic self-stimulatory behaviors that distracted other workers from their tasks. Several of the project subjects shout, scream, and laugh loudly. Would these behaviors be tolerated by other workers, or must they first be eliminated before the deaf-blind person can gain entry into subsidized employment?

Must adjustments in staff:worker ratios be made to accommodate deaf-blind rubella workers?
The greatest concern of STP staff regarding placement of deaf-blind rubella workers was that they would require an unreasonable amount of staff attention. This question and the question of communication skills were the two most significant issues related to the workshop's acceptance of deaf-blind workers.

The workshop targeted for placement was Olympus, which is considered an exemplary replication of the STP model. The site was fairly close to the homes of three of the deaf-blind students who lived in the Seattle area with family during summer vacation. Olympus agreed to provide space for three deaf-blind workers, but our project staff provided the necessary supervision and training, as well as the work tasks. The workshop was available for use five days each week for an eight-week period from mid-June to mid-August. The program was carried out with these three pupils for four days each week, from 9:30 a.m. to approximately 3:00 p.m. each day.

Subjects
Three severely retarded students deaf and blind due to rubella from the Washington State School for the Blind were chosen

because of their ages (approaching the final years of their public educations), their skill levels, and their summer residence with family in the Seattle area.

Subject 1. Subject 1 was a 19-year-old female with severe-to-profound hearing loss and severe visual impairment requiring special low vision spectacles that corrected to 20/80 for distance, but with a near acuity of three to four inches. This visual impairment, due to congenital rubella, was complicated or worsened by her tendency not to use her vision at all, which resulted in functional blindness at times. She had academic skills at the six-year level, could identify 23 capital letters, rote counted to 20, and had difficulty with balance, but had generally good finger and hand dexterity. She could perform five-part assemblies and could travel independently upon cue to the work room. She relied upon signs and gestures at the three-year level. She exhibited certain behaviors such as having tantrums when under pressure, and she was sometimes abusive to others. When working, she tended to move her hands in front of her face and filter light through her fingers. She tended to work very slowly, although she learned new tasks in two to four hours.

Subject 2. Subject 2 was a 17-year-old female with a severe-to-profound hearing loss and legal blindness due to congenital rubella. She wore cataract spectacles, used her right eye for critical seeing, and worked at a distance of three feet for near acuity. She suffered from scoliosis and heart defect, neither of which appeared to affect her school and vocational activities. Psychological testing showed a Letter Performance MA of 11 years. She had learned most skills up to age 6 years. She communicated by sign and gesture. Her greatest behavioral problem was perseveration, resulting in production rates between 10 percent and 15 percent.

Subject 3. Subject 3 was an 18-year-old male with total deafness and blindness due to congenital rubella. Developmental scores ranged from 0 to 84 months, with his lowest scores in the areas of language, and his highest scores in the areas of tactual perception. Prior to entering the project, he had learned to match shapes, do simple sorting, and complete several tasks independently. Incidents of aggression had occurred and he frequently emitted piercing screams, swung his head from side to side, hit his thighs with his forearms, and laughed loudly.

Subject 3 exhibited the screaming and laughing throughout the first year of vocational training, which covered one to two hours each school day. His finger and manual dexterity was readily apparent, and his aptitude for learning new assembly tasks was good. By the end of the first training session of 20 to 30 minutes, he usually showed signs of having learned the steps involved and could carry out the manipulations. Throughout his training, however, he would insert self-stimulatory behaviors (such as bringing parts to his lips, or retaining his hand in the parts bins and stirring the parts) that prevented him from reaching criteria.

Pretraining and placement

Two project staff members were available to work with the subjects at the workshop: one full-time and the other half-time. Both were doctoral students at the University of Washington and staff members of the project. To facilitate transition, all three subjects received training on two different assembly tasks for four weeks at the end of the school year, immediately prior to entering the workshop. The tasks chosen were designed to duplicate tasks found at Olympus, one being a duplication of a production task that was a part of subcontract work at the workshop. Other tasks duplicated those used for initial worker training. At the end of the pretraining period (carried out by peer tutors), the two female subjects had reached full proficiency on the two tasks, while the lower-functioning male subject had learned the basic steps but had incorporated self-stimulatory movements that required one-on-one staff supervision and training.

In order to introduce the subjects into the work environment in an orderly fashion, they were phased in, with the first worker on site for two weeks before the second worker was introduced. Then another two-week period elapsed before the third subject was introduced. Because of this lagged entry schedule, one subject was present for 8 full weeks, the second for 6 weeks, and the third (the lower-functioning subject) for 4 weeks.

The specific tasks on which the subjects were trained were bagging (two mechanical assemblies) (Figure 1); a cable harness assembly (Figure 2); and a circuit board assembly (Figure 3). Daily production records were maintained for all three subjects. Exact time spent on various jobs and numbers of units completed permitted exact calculation of wages. The workshop

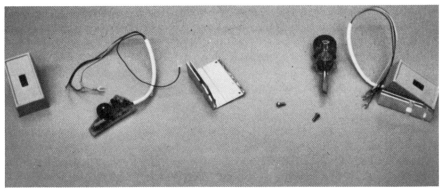

Figure 1. Task of bagging two mechanical assemblies.

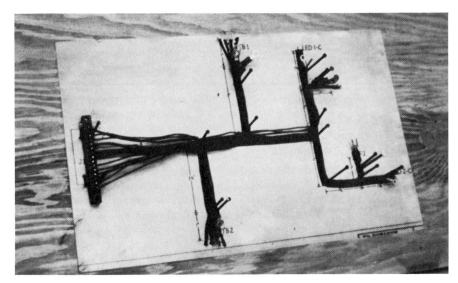

Figure 2. A cable harness assembly.

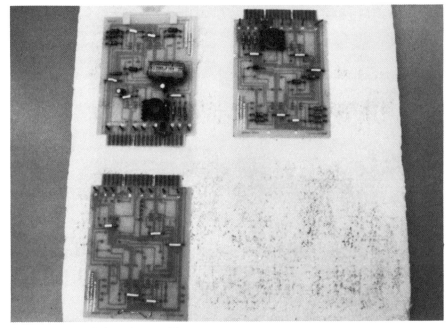

Figure 3. A circuit-board assembly.

had calculated production norms for all tasks used. Wages were paid to subjects by the project rather than by Olympus, but were computed according to Olympus standards, with each worker being paid exactly what would have been earned had he or she been an Olympus employee.

None of the subjects responded negatively to the new workshop placement, and all three carried out the assemblies at the level they had achieved at school before they were introduced to the work setting. Parts bins and reinforcement procedures in the classroom duplicated those at Olympus.

Results

Subject 1. Subject 1 had reached criterion on the pretraining tasks prior to entering the workshop. She missed no days of work (36 days total employment), worked a total of 120.5 hours, and earned $140.70. She reached criterion on one new task (TA-20, a small electronic assembly task), and was progressing on the cable harness task at the end of the workshop experience. While her production was clearly on par with many of the regular workshop employees, she worked slowly at times and did not respond to efforts to speed her work. She was also able to move independently from the workroom to the rest room and the eating area. She independently used the pop machine upon receiving the sign "break time," but did not return to work following her break without a cue. None of her work behaviors appeared to distract other workers, the only difficulty being that she sat in chairs that were regularly used by other workers.

At the end of her workshop experience, project staff and workshop staff agreed that subject 1 could likely fit in as a regular workshop employee in that setting and perform nonvisual tasks.

Subject 2. This subject attended work a total of 59.25 hours on 21 out of 31 days, earning $44.61. Her 50 percent absence rate was attributed to illness or tiredness by her family. Although efforts were made to interrupt her perseverating on steps by simply pointing to the next step in the sequence, those behaviors did not decrease during her workshop experience. Subject 2 had learned the pretrained tasks to proficiency level prior to starting her workshop experience. Upon entry into the workshop environment, she immediately resumed her performance on the two pretrained tasks. She also learned the

TA-20 assembly to criterion and started training in circuit-board stuffing. Again, her perseveration of steps greatly hindered her work performance, and her slow rate together with her frequent absences resulted in low earnings.

Project and workshop staff agreed that subject 2 could be considered an appropriate potential worker in the Olympus setting, although workshop staff had certain reservations that will be addressed later. Upon returning to her school program, efforts at eliminating or reducing her perseveration were begun, as this behavior was viewed as the only one that was preventing her from attaining higher productivity levels.

Subject 3. Upon entry to the workshop, this subject was quick to resume his training. His work behavior was somewhat erratic, with near-perfect assemblies on some days, but loss of sequence and frequent self-stimulatory behaviors on other days. Because of this erratic good-day/bad-day performance, it was necessary for a trainer to be close to him at the workshop at all times.

Subject 3 attended a total of 17 out of a possible 21 days. Absences were due to illness confirmed by the subject's family and accompanied by obvious symptoms. Subject worked a total of 50.5 hours and earned $43.35. The etiology of his erratic work behaviors was never discovered and they were never controlled. At the beginning of subject 3's work experience, his screams had little effect upon the regular Olympus workers. Near the end of the work experience, however, these screaming incidents escalated slightly, while the tolerance of the other workers seemed to decrease. As more and more regular Olympus workers became distracted and even alarmed by the screams, it became necessary to remove subject 3 from the work floor.

Overall, it was concluded by project staff and workshop staff that subject 3 did not have sufficient appropriate work and nonwork behaviors to fit into the workshop

setting. His failure to work consistently without error necessitated the constant presence of a trainer. The subject's heavy training and supervision needs, coupled with his distracting screams, were viewed as simply too difficult for workshop staff to accommodate. It should be noted, however, that in spite of the heavy training and supervision requirements, subject 3 earned close to the workshop average in wages, although his distracting behaviors clearly affected his work performance.

As a result of this work experience, it was concluded that school instructional programming should stress continued vocational training in the area of assembly and bagging, with efforts to eliminate the vocalizations and self-stimulatory behaviors that distracted other workers and prevented more efficient work performance.

Table 1 summarizes and compares the performances of three deaf-blind rubella workers to the severely handicapped workers at Olympus. It includes their monthly incomes, number of contacts per hour with supervisory staff, and production rates. Clearly, subject 1 performed at levels commensurate with those of Olympus workers. Subject 2 had lower wages and productivity rates than Olympus workers or subject 1, but her supervisory contacts were in the acceptable range. It is quite probable that increasing supervisory contacts would have brought subject 2's rates and wages up considerably. Subject 3 required considerably more supervisory contacts than Olympus workers, but was able to earn wages approaching the shop mean.

Conclusions

Our experience in the Olympus placement has led us to the following conclusions in regard to the four questions we initially raised.

Generalization of pretrained work skills and general work skills. The workshop placement involved a change of the students' daily routines (a one-hour car trip each morning and afternoon), a new

Table 1. Comparison of deaf-blind students to severely handicapped Olympus workers.

Subject	Monthly Income	Number of Contacts with Supervisor/Hour	Production Rate (percent)
1	85.00	4	28
2	37.00	5	18
3	51.00	18	21
Olympus workers	51.00[a]	5-7	NA[b]

[a]Mean wage of 18 workers over 8 months, range $30-$120.
[b]NA, not available.

work setting, new work stations (workbenches and stools rather than tables and chairs), and new trainers (project staff rather than regular teachers and peer tutors). Despite these changes, the subjects were able to carry over the pretrained tasks into the new setting. All three subjects quickly adjusted to the new work setting, and immediately began assembly sequences upon being given the parts. The two female subjects, who had enough vision for mobility and were more ambulatory, quickly learned the locations of the restroom and eating areas. The male subject, due to his total blindness and balance problems, was assisted in moving from one area to another. While staff believed that he could have learned to move independently about the workshop, the presence of dangerous machinery led us to decide not to attempt such training. Staff agreed that a single safe path would have sufficed for such training. The subjects' generalization was viewed as successful, with the pretraining on the tasks seen as valuable.

Communication skills required of staff. Because the emphasis of this project was on examining the feasibility of regular subsidized work programs for the deaf-blind, staff decided that fluency in signing would not be a requirement for trainers. The two project staff members who trained the three subjects did not sign. The teachers of the three subjects taught the project staff the few basic signs that the subjects knew. Staff attempted to sign as much as possible in order to elicit signed responses from the subjects. The most crucial communication occurred at the moment of task completion, when the worker was required to raise his or her hand, sign "finished" and "pay me." Physical cues rather than signed cues sufficed for most other transactions. At the end of the workshop program, project staff and workshop staff concluded that workers with this population could learn the requisite few signs without extensive training. Staff agreed that a fluent signer would be preferred so that more language learning could take place in the workplace. However, the lack of such a fluent signer seemed to place the deaf-blind worker at no greater disadvantage than the many severely retarded seeing and hearing workers who are nonverbal and learn by demonstration and physical assistance.

Self-stimulatory behaviors. One of our concerns was how other workers would react to the behaviors of the deaf-blind

workers. We found that their reactions varied. The two female subjects who had very limited but sufficient vision for movement about the workshop were quickly assimilated into the work force. Many of their off-task behaviors, such as perseveration, or filtering light through their fingers, were similar to behaviors exhibited by other workers. In social settings, such as at breaks and lunch, the sighted and hearing workers allowed these two subjects to sit and eat with them, the only problem arising when one of the subjects sat in a chair that was usually used by one of the other workers.

The behaviors of the third subject, however, were quite another matter. Over the course of his four-week placement, his screaming became more and more distracting to the other workers. While at first the other workers were able to continue working following his screams, as time progressed, workers became more and more agitated by his screams, until several workers walked off the workfloor. Another behavior that proved very disconcerting to the sighted workers was the subject's habit of reaching out and touching things and people around him. During lunch, he often reached out and touched the others around the table, and while being led off and onto the workfloor he extended his arms. This frightened some of the other workers, although their fear decreased as their exposure to his reaching behaviors increased. When the subject hit his thighs with his forearm, he did not seem to distract the other workers, as such self-stimulatory behaviors were occasionally seen on the floor anyway and are fairly typical self-stimulatory behaviors in severely retarded persons.

Both project and workshop staff concluded that subject 3's screaming would not be acceptable in that work setting, and must be eliminated prior to any placement in a work setting such as Olympus.

Staff:worker ratios. Here again, program staff estimates of ideal staff:worker ratios differed according to the individual subjects' performance. As noted above, Olympus staff accepted the two female subjects, who were not distracting, who learned new tasks readily, and who were able to work without supervision. The fact that their production was slow and needed improvement was not a new problem in this setting, and would be typical in most workshops. These subjects' independence in toileting, taking breaks, lunch, and production was seen as adequate for entry

into the subsidized employment setting. However, Olympus staff continued to express some doubts about working with even these high-functioning deaf-blind workers. Upon being pressed by project staff to estimate their ability to place these workers, Olympus staff stated that one or two workers of this higher functioning level could be admitted to the workshop setting, but additional staff might be required initially to supervise them.

Project staff members do not agree with the workshop staff on this issue. In our view, these two deaf-blind workers performed at a level equal to or higher than most of the other workers, and presented training problems no different from those of the other severely retarded workers. Two reasons for this difference in opinion present themselves: 1) during the summer placement, workshop staff were very busy training their workers on new tasks associated with several new subcontracts and therefore never directly worked with or spent time observing these subjects; and 2) workshop staff relied upon verbal "callouts" to reinforce on-task behaviors. Staff often called out praise of good work behaviors. Naturally, deaf-blind workers cannot be reinforced in this manner. Alternative reinforcement schemes would require hands-on work with deaf-blind workers by workshop staff. Although the verbal "callouts" are not appropriate for deaf-blind workers, workshop trainers and supervisory staff might adjust their workfloor supervision in order to remain closer to the deaf-blind workers to deliver physical reinforcements.

Future efforts
The results of this project indicate that the deaf-blind rubella students are capable of performing work tasks in a subsidized work environment for the severely handicapped. They are able to perform not only at acceptable productivity levels, but also within acceptable rates of supervisory contacts. Both project and workshop staff agreed that at least some deaf-blind rubella workers could be assimilated into the Olympus program.

Given the range of functional levels present in the population of deaf-blind individuals, it would seem to be inappropriate to attempt to make any vocational decisions based upon generalized norms for this group. While two of the subjects in this project were found to be acceptable as workers in a subsidized work program, one was found to need additional training before being able to attend such a program. The findings of this project point out the need for individually determined vocational placements for deaf-blind students. Any attempts to develop vocational placements for these students as a group will undoubtedly result in inappropriate placements for some. The same range of options available to other severely handicapped persons for vocational placement should be available for deaf-blind rubella workers. Further, it seems likely that at least some of these deaf-blind rubella students can be served in subsidized work programs that already exist for persons with severe handicaps.

References

Bellamy, G.T., Horner, R.H., & Inman, D.P. (1979). *Vocational habilitation of severely retarded adults: A direct service technology.* Baltimore: University Park Press.

Bellamy, G.T., Borbeau, P.E., & Sowers, J. (1983). Work and work-related services:Postsched options. In M. Snell (ed.), *Systematic instruction of the moderately and severely handicapped* (2nd ed.). Columbus, OH: Charles E. Merrill.

Groht, M. (1958). *Natural language for deaf children.* Washington, DC: Volta Bureau.

Mitaug, D.E., Hagmier, L.D., & Haring, N.G. (1977). The relationship between training activities and job placement in vocational education of the severely and profoundly handicapped. *American Association for the Education of the Severely and Profoundly Handicapped Review,* **2,** 25-45.

Romer, L.T. (1983). Vocational module development for deaf-blind severely retarded secondary students. Manuscript submitted for publication.

Van Uden, A. (1970). *A world of language for deaf children.* Rotterdam, The Netherlands: Rotterdam University Press.

Wilcox, B. & Bellamy, G.T. (1982). *Design of high school programs for severely handicapped students.* Baltimore: Paul H. Brookes.

Dennis G. Busse, Lyle T. Romer, doctoral candidates; Rebecca R. Fewell, Ph.D., professor; College of Education, University of Washington at Seattle; Patricia F. Vadasy, M.P.H., research publications editor for the experimental education unit at the Child Development & Mental Retardation Center, University of Washington, Seattle, WA 98195.

Group Homes for Severely Multiply Handicapped Persons with Visual Problems

L. Guldager; M. Hamill; R. D. McGlamery

Abstract: Argues that community residences for small groups of people, and the provision of day activity programs designed to increase functional levels, is the only viable, humane alternative to institutionalization of severely multiply handicapped persons with visual problems. Living in a highly structured home environment where individual needs are addressed by caring and qualified staff can and should be provided to those without self-preservation skills. Opportunities to participate in suitable prevocational activities are also necessary. The cost of such programs is the same as for institutional care, and funding can be secured.

The establishment of community group homes for severely multiply handicapped persons is slowly becoming a reality in Connecticut. It requires a philosophical commitment as well as a practical commitment of energy, resourcefulness, planning, dedication and funds. It is an idea whose time has come; in fact, it is long overdue. There is cause for cautious optimism among those who are steadfastly proceeding toward the attainment of this type of supervised lifetime placement for all people who need it.

In recent years, there have been significant improvements in the quality and diversity of needed programs and services for severely multiply handicapped children in private residential settings. Parents, educators and representatives of various social service agencies have unrelentingly championed the cause of all handicapped people. They have been the impetus behind the legislation of the 1960s and 1970s passed by the U.S. Congress, interpreted, promulgated and monitored on the state level, and implemented within specific program settings. The results, as observed in the program at the Oak Hill School in Hartford, Connecticut, have been earlier identification and diagnosis, better referral networks, education and training programs

Presented at American Foundation for the Blind's 1982 Helen Keller Seminar on "Standards and Models for Excellence," October 28, 1982.

tailored to individual needs, more appropriate and specialized medical and dental treatment, and ongoing therapeutic services. For moderately affected, higher functioning adults, greater opportunities for remunerative employment are available.

Even more recently, opportunities for living with dignity and purpose in a normal environment have been afforded to an increasing number of people who are multiply impaired but capable of functioning successfully in supervised group home and workshop settings.

As plans continue to be developed and implemented for community-based living, learning and working programs for moderately affected multiply handicapped persons, and as the national trend toward deinstitutionalization continues to gain momentum, we are faced with the prospect of institutions and nursing homes filled with severely and profoundly multiply handicapped adults, many of whom have functional visual problems. After many years in publicly funded school programs, severely multiply handicapped persons are relegated, at the age of 21, to lifetime environments which, in our judgment, are totally unacceptable and reflect lack of foresight and innovation. It is our contention that community residences and day activity centers designed to improve functional levels can and should be provided regardless of the number, complexity and severity of handicapping conditions. Following is a discussion of some of the major issues involved in creating community homes and programs for disabled populations, as illustrated by different Oak Hill models.

Self-preservation skills essential

When planning group homes for multiply handicapped persons, a primary determination must be made. Do the prospective residents have self-preservation skills? That is, are they capable of reacting appropriately to an actual or potential life-threatening danger? For example, would potential residents promptly leave a dwelling when the audio/visual fire alarm is activated, or when told to do so by a staff member? Would they respond to procedures and routines carried out consistently and repetitively during emergency drills? Can they be depended upon not to jump out a third-story window?

Assuming that prospective group home members do have such self-prservation skills, the dwelling in which they will live must meet applicable fire and safety code regulations. Among the major requirements are:

• for a multi-level dwelling, two enclosed staircases leading directly to the front and back outside exits;

• fire-rated furnace enclosure;

• fire-rated carpets;

• fire/smoke detection system;

• elimination of all dead-bolt locks;

• fire alarm system hooked into the local fire station; and

• self-closing fire doors in the kitchen area.

Oak Hill opened its first off-campus group home in February, 1978. A married couple lived in the residence, which housed seven visually impaired teenage girls, some of whom had part-time jobs in the community. Upon completion of the school program, some obtained competitive employment; others were placed in a sheltered workshop program and remained in the group home as adult residents.

Since 1978, our school population has changed. Now, all of our students are severely multiply handicapped. As they become more proficient in everyday life skills and as their behaviors become more socially acceptable, they are housed in facilities that provide them with greater opportunities for skill development and maintenance. Although the programs remain highly structured, there is a progressive shift toward greater normalization. By the time the students reach adulthood, they are already familiar with a group home environment and routine.

For this reason, the transition from a student home to an adult residence is less traumatic.

For the purposes of normalization, a group home for four to eight residents located in a suburb, yet within leisurely walking distance of a large shopping area, is ideal. The Newington Group Home, which accommodates seven adults, is a good example. Established and conducted by the Connecticut Institute for the Blind, it is the first group home in Connecticut for multiply handicapped adults, all of whom are visually impaired. The spacious Victorian-style home was renovated to comply with the aforementioned fire regulations in 1980. In addition to upgrading plumbing and electrical systems, a small wood-frame addition was erected to provide more bedrooms and one more bathroom. The layout of the second floor was modified to grant easier maneuverability to the residents. Attention was also given to providing an up-to-date, functional kitchen with abundant cabinet space.

In August, 1981, Thompson House in Newington was ready for occupancy. Six women and one man moved into the residence within the first few weeks. Of the seven adults, who range in age from 21 to 39 years, four are totally blind and three are legally blind. All have deficits in intellectual functioning ranging from borderline to moderate retardation. Three have gross motor problems. Associated health problems include obesity, partial hearing loss, and migraine headaches.

During the first few months, emphasis was placed on orienting each adult to the spacious house and to the immediate environs. Also, special attention was given to kitchen facilities. Individual problems such as personal hygiene, dining etiquette, and time management were identified and addressed simultaneously in order to eliminate, or at least mitigate, any irritations which could cause friction among the residents.

Relationships among the Thompson House family members are positive and mutually supportive. Group activities such as holiday parties, cookouts for families and friends, and trips to the movies generate a spirit of comraderie. Based on their own interests, as well as suggestions from staff, house members also engage in individual or small group activities. Sometimes, residents participate in events with people from other organizations, as when three adults joined the cast of a musical production spon-

sored by another private agency serving handicapped persons. Since private transportation services are available, the adults are able to attend many events in the community. In addition, as a result of extensive orientation and mobility training, two residents are capable of traveling independently to nearby shops.

Opportunities to explore the community are enhanced because of proximity to shops and other much-frequented establishments where items may be purchased and services obtained. A movie theater, public swimming pool, and public transportation are readily accessible. Learning experiences and supervised leisure time pursuits involving community interaction abound in this setting. Individual program plans designed to promote skill proficiency and normalization are written, reviewed and regularly revised by staff.

An integral component of the total Newington Program is a meaningful, productive work program. All the residents have acquired a reasonable degree of vocational skill competency and have met or exceeded minimum standards for acceptable social behavior. All attend a nearby sheltered workshop which is conducted by the state agency for the blind. One especially skilled and productive resident receives the minimum wage for work performed; others are engaged in piecework projects and can earn up to one-half the minimum wage. Earnings are determined according to a preestablished formula that is based on such factors as the complexity of the job performed and the number of "finished products" completed. Both programs are conducted in accordance with federal and state regulations. Twenty-five percent of a resident's income, which consists primarily of wages and social security income, is paid toward the rent. Other necessary services are paid for according to a sliding scale fee.

Needs of the more impaired adult

Thus far, we have focused on persons with self-preservation skills. But what happens to persons without these abilities—those who are severely and profoundly multiply handicapped and visually impaired? For the purpose of our discussion, a severely and profoundly impaired person is defined as an individual having some or all of these disabilities in varying degrees: visual, speech or hearing deficits; orthopedic handicaps; neurological disorders; emotional disturbance; learning disabilities; and functional severe or profound mental retardation. Additional

medical problems, such as heart disease and diabetes, may require treatment and monitoring. Inappropriate social behavior and severe "acting out" are other serious problems that must be addressed.

The current Oak Hill population of 212 students ranges in age from 2 to 21 years. All are multiply handicapped and visually impaired. While extensive programs for this population have long been available, at the age 21, after numerous years of these mandated programs, the severely impaired adult has limited options—none of which are appropriate. The unacceptable choices are institutions or nursing homes—for life. In any case, individual programs to address specific needs, provide required ancillary services, guarantee consistent therapeutic treatment, maintain existing daily living skill competency and, to prevent regression, will either cease to exist or are minimal *at best*.

Is group home placement and a day activity program a feasible alternative? Some professionals maintain that, because of the multiplicity and complexity of handicapping conditions, no further substantial gains can be made. Therefore, they argue, there is little justification for community placement when existing institutions will provide custodial care. Parents are anxious about severing ties with a self-contained facility and program where there are numerous trained staff and reliable, proven backup systems in place. If serious medical problems requiring daily medication and close observation exist, there are additional real concerns related to treatment and control. Surely, these are legitimate concerns, but when we consider the alternatives, community placement is the most viable, growth-promoting solution.

Establishing community residences

Securing a community residence for severely multiply handicapped persons without self-preservation skills was not an easy task. The selection of the land sites and community was accomplished after much research. Special permission from the local zoning board was required. In accordance with the law, a public hearing was held and town residents were invited to attend and voice any concerns. Since Oak Hill School is a long-established service agency that is well-known throughout Connecticut, opposition to the establishment of group homes *per se* in this town was virtually nonexistent. Those anxieties the community did have centered for the most part on the exteriors of the proposed homes. Would they have an institutional look? Other concerns focused on the residents, the staff, and the adequacy of supervision. The school's superintendent addressed all of these matters and explained the total program in detail, successfully assuaging these apprehensions.

The dwelling had to be in compliance with the Life Safety Code, making renovation of an existing house nearly impossible and leaving new construction the most workable solution. Constructing a home which is aesthetically pleasing, provides standard creature comforts, and yet incorporates the stringent fire and safety features required for this type of structure, was viewed as the most appropriate direction to take. With the assistance of an architectural firm, we were able to design and construct two such homes in Granby, Connecticut. To the best of our knowledge, these community residences are the first group homes in the country built exclusively to the specifications of the Life Safety Code for the purpose of housing severely to profoundly multiply impaired persons who lack self-preservation skills.

In addition to the previously noted safeguards, the houses provide:
• complete fire/smoke detection and alarm system which is connected to the local fire station;
• extra large bedroom windows with horizontal sliding glass which can be used as emergency exits;
• flame-resistant lumber;
• fireproof floor structure because the dwelling is constructed on a grade-level concrete slab (no crawl space);
• no duct work throughout the home;
• wide, strategically located doors leading directly to outside (no stairs);
• fire-barrier walls;
• special heating and cooling systems which are fire-resistant;
• fire-rated doors on kitchen and utility room housing the furnace;
• a staff room whose location and design allow direct observation of residents in common living areas at all times; and
• light beam alarms that emit sounds when activated by persons entering and leaving the homes.

The two homes, within a block of each other, are nestled in a suburban area of one-family homes, about three miles from the center of town. Since the residents are not capable of availing themselves of community resources independently, it was not necessary for the homes to be near a shopping center or mass transportation system.

The residences are single-story homes of contemporary design and have approximately 3,500 square feet of living space. Each accommodates six adults who have individual bedrooms and share three full bathrooms. The fully equipped kitchens, which contain laundry areas, were built to provide easy access and maneuverability to persons in wheelchairs. The same holds true for the bathrooms, which have shower stalls four feet wide and other safety devices. The dining room and living room are adjacent to the kitchen and provide access, via sliding glass doors, to the patio. All bedrooms converge onto a large family room with a cathedral ceiling and provisions for considerable natural light. In addition to staff and storage rooms, there is an additional bedroom and bath, designated for arts and crafts projects and indoor games.

Educational programs

Each resident has an individual program plan which specifies the objectives to be reached within a predetermined time frame and activities designed to facilitate their achievement. Maintenance and ongoing reinforcement of existing skills are addressed. Emphasis in the home program is placed on teaching daily living skills, personal and rudimentary household management, and various forms of communication skills, acceptable behavior, and leisure time activities. Individual behavior modification programs, including time-out procedures, have been developed in detail and are implemented as the need arises by trained staff.

The program also allows for imagination and innovation in the pursuit of the least restrictive, most normalizing environment. Although the residents are low functioning, they can take advantage of public offerings such as open air concerts, community firework displays, parades and fairs. Field trips to public wading pools, parks and picnic areas can also be fun experiences. Other outdoor seasonal activities include running under the backyard sprinkler, walking in leaves, and, in the winter months, playing in the snow and sledding. Riding adult-sized three-wheel bicycles provides residents with additional opportunities to develop gross motor skills in the fresh air, and parallel bars provide the physically impaired resident with much-needed exercises. Although the entire program is highly structured, there is considerable flexibility in carrying out normal activities that have been adapted to the needs of the handicapped.

As shown in Tables 1 and 2, the staffing pattern in each home provides for adequate supervision at all times. In each residence, one teacher and two assistant teachers for each shift (day and evening) conduct the living and day activity programs. They are assisted by an instructor who divides her time between the two groups of residents. One child care worker is awake and on duty during the night hours. In the event of staff absences, replacement personnel from Oak Hill School are readily available.

Crucial to the entire program is the day activity component conducted in a rented facility located close by. In accordance

Table 1. Thompson House staffing pattern for seven residents.

Position	Days	Time	Total Hours per Week
Group home supervisor	Monday & Wednesday	Flexible	22½
Resident home services worker[a]	Monday—Friday	6:30 A.M.- 8:30 P.M.	
	Monday—Friday	3:00 P.M.- 9:00 P.M.	40
Home services worker	Wednesday—Friday	7:00 P.M.- 9:30 A.M.	
	Saturday & Sunday	7:00 P.M.- 3:00 P.M.	23½
Home services worker	Monday & Tuesday	7:00 A.M.- 9:30 P.M.	
	Saturday & Sunday	7:00 A.M.- 3:00 P.M.	21
Home services worker	Monday—Friday	2:00 P.M.-10:00 P.M.	40
Home services worker	Saturday & Sunday	2:00 P.M.-10:00 P.M.	16
Homes services worker	Friday	10:00 P.M.- 7:00 A.M.	
	Saturday	2:00 P.M.-10:00 P.M.	
	Sunday	10:00 P.M.- 7:00 A.M.	26
Home services worker	Sunday	2:00 P.M.-10:00 P.M.	8

[a]On call during the night

Table 2. Juniper Group Home staffing pattern for six residents.

Position	Days	Time	Total Hours per Week
Teacher	5—Flexible	Flexible	35
Instructor	2½—Flexible	Flexible	18¾
Assistant teacher	Sunday—Thursday	7:00 A.M.- 3:00 P.M.	37½
Assistant teacher	Sunday—Thursday	3:00 P.M.-11:00 P.M.	37½
Assistant teacher	Tuesday—Saturday	7:00 A.M.- 3:00 P.M.	37½
Assistant teacher	Tuesday—Saturday	3:00 P.M.-11:00 P.M.	37½
Night child care worker	Sunday—Thursday	11:00 P.M.- 7:00 A.M.	40
Weekend child care worker	Sunday & Monday	3:00 P.M.-11:00 P.M.	15
Weekend night child care worker	Friday & Saturday	11:00 P.M.- 7:00 A.M.	16

with principles of normalization, day activity takes place in a site outside the residence from Monday through Friday, approximating the typical workday for most nonhandicapped people. Staff who work with the adults in the group homes also conduct the day program.

Since the residents do not have the capabilities necessary for participating in workshop activities, they engage in pre-vocational types of activities consistent with their individual functioning levels. These include: stuffing envelopes, folding paper, stapling papers together, using paper clips to secure papers, using fixed-size wrenches for assembling purposes, and sorting by color, shape, size and/or texture. Each client's job is task-analyzed and usually differs from that of his peers because of individual differences. Work tolerance ranges from 30 seconds to 15 minutes and allowances for frequent breaks are made. Rolling about on mats, playing on outdoor swings and monkey bars, walking about, playing with soft balls, and other diversionary activities are forms of tension release. Behavior modification techniques, tailored to the individual, are also reinforced in this setting. An adult is rewarded for good work and behavior by being allowed to play with a favorite object, walk about, roll on mats, or do whatever has been identified as pleasurable. Time-out procedures are also carried out when "acting out" or other types of severe unacceptable behaviors are manifested.

Staff training

Initial and ongoing staff training is crucial to the success of any community-based residence program for severely impaired persons. Those who work directly with this population need a wide variety of specialized skills, knowledge, and competencies in order to be effective. In addition to requiring that prospective direct care staff have prior experience (paid or volunteer) in working with handicapped persons, Oak Hill provides a comprehensive training program which is coordinated by a full-time staff development specialist.

Prior to actual on-the-job experience, new staff participate in two days of pre-service orientation. Topics include: major program goals and objectives, an overview of the multiply handicapped person, and the importance of the team approach. Those aspects of direct care which are critical to the health and safety of the clients are introduced at this time and addressed in more detail during subsequent sessions. They include: basic first aid, the Heimlich maneuver, mouth-to-mouth resuscitation, lifting and transferring non-ambulatory persons, basic behavior modification, basic sign language, and emergency procedures. The coordinator of nursing services explains any specific known medical problems of the residents and trains the staff to perform needed procedures such as urine testing and insulin injections for diabetics. General policies, procedures and related information are comprehensively delineated in a staff manual provided to each employee.

A second training component consists of regularly scheduled and "as needed" consultations with specialists in medicine, physical and occupational therapy, nutrition, social services, orientation and mobility, and behavior modification with staff at Oak Hill School. Although supportive services are community-based, all of the resources and expertise of the school

are available to the group home staff. In addition to assessing client needs and providing appropriate program suggestions, these specialists are also responsible for periodic monitoring. This multidisciplinary approach assures the well-being of the adults being served.

In-depth training characterizes the third component of staff development. Analysis of the results of staff needs-assessment surveys determines the subject areas to be addressed over a period of 12 months. The staff development specialist coordinates the course offerings, which usually include cardiopulmonary resuscitation (CPR), sign language (beginner and advanced), effects of medication, seizures, language development, infection control, writing and implementing effective individual program plans, diseases of the eyes, and specific disabilities such as cerebral palsy, mental retardation, and deafness, among others.

The fourth component focuses on the need to grow professionally by reading relevant publications that are centrally located in the Oak Hill staff library, taking field trips to other programs that serve the handicapped, attending and participating in appropriate workshops and conferences, and taking courses offered at local colleges and universities.

Another facet of staff training that involves adult group home staff, addresses effective communication and public relations with neighbors and town residents. This topic is covered in depth prior to group home occupancy. Our past experiences in establishing friendly relationships with the community have been quite effective. A month after our Granby Group Homes were occupied, an open house was held for neighbors. They were able to tour the facilities, meet staff, ask questions, and voice concerns. By taking the initiative and "reaching out" with openness and friendship, we elicited positive responses from many neighbors. Local church groups purchased Christmas trees and assisted in decorating them. Other local residents suggested landscape revisions and volunteered to plant shrubs, bushes and flowers. Some neighboring farmers have donated produce from their gardens. Occasionally, area children have visited and brought homemade cookies to the residents. Others have dropped by in the evening to assist with planned activities. Staff have taken clients into the community to local grocery stores, drug stores, and public parks. In addition to introducing the adults to a variety of normalizing activities and events, the trips also afford the townspeople opportunities to observe the adults and, we hope, to initiate interaction.

Funding

Our final concern is funding, a source of concern during the best of times and an ever present stumbling block during these periods of austerity and tight fiscal management. It is important to note, however, that *the group home and day activity programs we advocate cost the same as those programs involving institutionalization.*

Several funding sources do exist. Government support is available from Intermediate Care Facilities for the Mentally Retarded (ICF/MR) and other entitlement programs. In more recent years, the U.S. Department of Housing and Urban Development has appropriated funds under Section 202, Section 8, and a Congregate Living Program has expanded possibilities for securing federal assis-

tance. The Farmers Home Project also makes public monies available, but only to rural areas.

Syndication is yet another alternative, a concept that is getting more and more popular for private investors as a tax shelter. Of course, there is still the conventional bank mortgage.

At present, The Connecticut Institute for the Blind has six group homes for students attending Oak Hill School; one adult group home in Newington for handicapped persons who are engaged in remunerative workshop programs; and two adult residences in Granby for severely multiply handicapped adults who attend a day activity program. Two additional group homes, identical to those in Granby, will be built in Glastonbury for occupancy by September, 1983. Our projections for 1996 include 28 *additional* community residences throughout Connecticut for persons with multiple impairments. Day activity programs will be "in place" for all residents.

Conclusion

Our experience with and knowledge of persons with a multiplicity of severe disabilities have guided our endeavors. Our research into, and personal observation of, life in large institutions have strongly reinforced our thinking. To languish in a custodial care environment without appropriate training programs, without an adequate number of well-trained staff, without opportunities to maintain learned skills and behaviors and to improve functional levels, is to exist in a subhuman environment conducive to regression. The only viable, positive, progressive alternative is an appropriate community residence and day activity program.

Lars Guldager, Ph.D., superintendent, Mary Hamill, M.A., assistant to the superintendent, Rebecca D. McGlamery, Ph.D., assistant superintendent, Oak Hill School, 120 Holcomb Street, Hartford, Connecticut 06112.

Perceptions of a Community Program for Multiply Handicapped Blind Young Adults

J. Syme; K. Wilton

Abstract: This article reports the results of a survey of the perceptions of parents of nine multiply handicapped young adults enrolled in a community living program in New Zealand and of the nine staff members who were working with the young adults. All the parents believed that the program had benefited their multiply handicapped children. Both parents and staff members strongly supported the involvement of parents in the program and the content and focus of the program. Although both the parents and the staff members believed that available support services were adequate, the social worker and adult rehabilitation services were viewed much less favorably by the parents than by the staff.

The role of parents in the education of handicapped children has changed considerably in the past few decades (Sarason & Doris, 1979). Not too long ago, parents often were viewed by professionals as scapegoats and identified as a major cause of their handicapped child's problems. In time, parents became politically involved in seeking the provision of better education for their children and, in some parts of the world, they have begun to participate as paraprofessionals in their children's educational programs (Kirk & Gallagher, 1983).

Although the close involvement of parents and professionals in the education of blind and visually impaired children has traditionally been advocated, such involvement has generally been difficult to achieve in the case of blind children with multiple handicaps. Such children are conspicuously few in number and usually attend residential schools, where they receive economically feasible special instruction in relation to their blindness (especially Braille reading and mobility training) and additional handicaps. Clearly, their parents have fewer oppor-

The authors wish to thank the Royal New Zealand Foundation for the Blind for its help with the survey. Special thanks also are due to the parents of the young adults and the staff of the Community Living Program, who made this study possible. Copies of the interview forms may be obtained on request from the authors.

tunities than do the parents of blind children who live at home to become involved in their education. In these circumstances, the concerns and perceptions of parents could well be different from those of the staff who work with the children, and it would be easy for the parents' views and concerns regarding their children's education to be overlooked. Similar difficulties would seem likely to arise vis-à-vis the postschool programs in which these children participate.

Little has been written about the education or postschool adjustment of multiply handicapped blind children in New Zealand, and no studies done in New Zealand have been published in this area. The brief survey reported in this article was conducted as a first step in this direction. It investigated the perceptions of the parents of multiply handicapped blind young adults who were enrolled in the Community Living Program— the major rehabilitation program for multiply handicapped blind young adults in New Zealand, as well as the staff employed in the program.

Community Living Program
The Community Living Program was established by the Royal New Zealand Foundation for the Blind to provide training in daily living and vocational skills for young blind adults with additional handicaps. The ultimate aim of the program is to integrate these young adults into the community by providing individualized train-

ing and support that will eventually enable them to live as independently as possible with support applicable to their needs.

At the time of the study, the young adults were living either in a semihostel residential facility or in a newly established family home, situated within the foundation complex, or at home (from which they commuted daily to the workshops and community living program); these were the only options available to them when they left school. All, however, received intensive training in the family home during the day on a 1-to-1 or 1-to-2 basis. The trainees were taken from the workshops at specific times to work on the skills they required for independence. For example, they were assessed in such daily living skills as doing laundry, cooking, and paying rent and budgeting. Most of them had limited mobility training or social and recreational experiences during their school years. Accordingly, the program emphasized these important skills that are required for the initiation and maintenance of relationships, the ability to react appropriately in social situations, and the utilization of recreational activities in the community. In the initial stages of the program, for instance, the participants would be encouraged to invite family members and friends to the family home for a meal, to participate in indoor bowling on the grounds, and to learn the route to the local store. In most cases, the participants were unable to perform these tasks at the beginning of the program.

The parents of these young blind adults had to come to terms with the change of philosophy engendered by the Community Living Program. Previous services had focused primarily on looking after handicapped persons, whereas the main emphasis of the Community Living Program was to teach them to take maximum responsibility for their lives and to increase their independence in the community. This change in emphasis aroused real concerns in some parents for the safety and general well-being of their children. The study was thus designed to examine the parents' and staff's perceptions of the newly formed Community Living Program and its effect on the young adults and their thoughts about other possible options for these young adults with regard to residence and vocation.

Subjects
The subjects were four fathers and five mothers of nine multiply handicapped blind young adults and the staff who were

attached to the training center attended by the young adults. The age range of the parents was 37-65 years (M = 50 years) and of the young adults 18-30 years (M = 24 years). All the young adults (six men and three women) had previously attended a residential school for blind or visually impaired children. Six of the nine young adults were totally blind, one had light perception only, and the remaining two had a limited degree of object perception.

Their additional handicaps varied widely and included physical disabilities (such as epilepsy or cardiac and respiratory conditions), hearing impairments, and speech impairments. At the time of the study, two of the young adults lived at home, three lived in a semihostel residential facility, and four lived in a family home administered by the Royal New Zealand Foundation for the Blind. The nine staff members (five men and four women, who ranged in age from 23-51 years with a mean of 37.8 years) were attached to the Community Living Program administered by the foundation.

Four of the staff (all men) were workshop supervisors; the remainder were involved in teaching and in the residential aspects of the program.

Procedure

Two brief, structured interview forms were developed for the study—one for the parents and one for the staff. All parents and staff members had previously been sent a letter inviting them to participate in the study, and all had agreed to participate. The parents were interviewed at home and the program staff were interviewed during working hours. Data were gathered on the attitudes of the parents and staff members toward the Community Living Program, including parental participation in the program, and on their perceptions of the adequacy of the services that were being provided.

Results

Parents' views

The parents were asked to rate the capabilities of their children in comparison to those of sighted persons of equivalent age on a 5-point scale (5 = very capable, 4 = capable, 3 = average, 2 = limited, and 1 = very limited). The mean ratings for work (1.78), independence in daily living activities (2.22), recreation management (2.22), organization of personal activities (1.88), and interpersonal skills (2.11) indicate that, in general, the parents believed

their children to have limited capabilities in these areas. However, six of the nine parents believed that their children had become noticeably more independent and better able to communicate since they left school. All the parents strongly wanted their children to make further progress, and all regarded the Community Living Program as having made an important contribution to their progress thus far. Seven of the nine parents strongly supported (and desired) parental involvement in the program and in decisions regarding their children and believed that they were more involved in their children's education and training now than they had been during the school years.

All the parents were concerned about future employment opportunities for their children and about their children's lack of independence in recreational pursuits. All except one parent believed that sheltered workshops were the most appropriate avenue of employment, though all the parents expressed a strong desire for more positive attitudes towards handicapped people by employers and for better training opportunities so that their children might eventually be able to obtain some form of open employment and achieve a degree of independence in community living and recreational activities.

Staff's attitudes

The staff members were asked to rate the adequacy of the various aspects of the Community Living Program in relation to the special educational needs of the participants. Their ratings were done on a 5-point scale from 5 (very adequate) to 1 (totally inadequate), and the mean ratings for the staff on the various aspects of the program were as follows: teaching = daily living skills (3.00), fostering independence (2.89), fostering socialization (2.67), and fostering recreational skills (3.00). These results indicate that the staff generally believed the program to be adequate. Seven of the nine staff members were strongly in favor of parents being involved in the program as members of the program team. The remaining two staff members believed that the presence of parents would diminish the young adults' opportunities to achieve independence.

The staff's views on appropriate employment options for the participants were consistent with those of the parents. Seven of the nine staff members believed that sheltered employment was the most appropriate option, although they did not rule out the possibility of eventual outside

employment after training for one or two of the participants.

Ratings of support services

Both the parents and the staff members were asked to rate the adequacy of available support services associated with the program. Support from social workers was perceived less favorably by the parents than by the staff (M for parents = 1.71, M for staff = 3.11; $t(16)$ = 2.53, $p < .03$), as was support from adult rehabilitation services (M for parents = 1.75, M for staff = 3.11; $t(16) = 2.53$, $p < .03$). However, the two groups were not dissimilar in relation to support from psychologists (M for parents = 2.17, M for staff = 3.33; $t(16) = 1.25$, $p < .24$), support from workshop staff (M for parents = 3.22, M for staff = 3.25; $t(16) = 0.06$, $p < .96$), and support from hostel staff (M for parents = 2.75, M for staff = 2.71; $t(16) = 0.07$, $p < .95$). These results indicate that although both groups viewed the support services as adequate, the parents thought these services (especially social work and rehabilitation services) to be less helpful than did the staff. A closer look at these particular support services and their relationship to the participants and their families thus seems warranted.

Postscript

Since the study was conducted, the program has grown and the participants now live in houses in the community. A vocational lunch scheme, which is maintained by trainees in the program, has been established at the foundation. Some trainees recently participated in the Outward-Bound Scheme—an outdoor residential program (based in the South Island) that is widely used by young adults from all over New Zealand. The program, which includes such activities as camping and sailing, is intended to build self-confidence and to foster cooperative skills and attitudes.

References

Kirk, S.A., & Gallagher, J.J. (1983). *Educating exceptional children* (4th ed.). Boston: Houghton-Mifflin Co.

Sarason, S.B., & Doris, J. (1979). *Educational handicap, public policy, and social history*. New York: Free Press.

Jenny Syme, B.A., Dip. Occup. Therapy, postgraduate student, Department of Education; Keri Wilton, Ph.D., senior lecturer in education, University of Auckland, Private Bag, Auckland 1, New Zealand.

Use of General Case Instruction with Visually Impaired, Multiply Handicapped Adults in the Sorting of National Zip Codes

W.W. Woolcock; M.B. Lengel

Abstract: The purpose of the study was to determine whether the acquisition of independent sorting skills on a representative sample of the first two digits in national zip codes (zip code prefixes) results in generalized independent sorting of all 100 national zip code prefixes. It was found that two of the three visually impaired, mentally retarded subjects demonstrated improved generalized performance on probes of their nontrained ability to sort 100 national zip code prefixes during and following instruction on 9 representative prefixes.

The recent emphasis on developing efficient strategies to teach individuals with severe handicaps to perform functional tasks across an array of instructional stimuli has included the selection of teaching materials that contain examples of the characteristics of all the possible stimuli involved in performing a particular generalized task. By selecting representative teaching materials, a general case response (Horner, Sprague, & Wilcox, 1982) may be taught so that "after instruction on some tasks in a particular class, any task in that class may be performed correctly" (Becker & Engelmann, 1978, p. 325). The objective of general case instruction, therefore, is to teach generalized responses that are reliably performed on a larger number of stimulus examples than are provided during instruction. Thus, general case instruction may increase instructional efficiency because teachers provide instruction only in the representative examples, rather than in all possible examples, particularly in cases such as the U.S. zip code prefixes 00 to 99, in which a great number of stimulus examples are presented.

The initial step in developing a general case response requires the definition of the "instructional universe" (Horner, Sprague, & Wilcox, 1982, p. 74) of all the possible stimulus conditions under which the target behavior will be performed. A minimum number of teaching examples is selected from this instructional universe to sample the full range of stimuli present in all the targeted stimulus examples. These selected teaching examples are sequenced in instructional sessions until the students attain a prespecified criterion level, following which the students are typically administered probe measures of their ability to perform, untrained, on the remaining examples in the instructional universe (see Horner, & McDonald, 1982).

General case instruction has been used successfully to teach a variety of generalized responses in vocational (Horner, & McDonald, 1982) and community settings (Horner, Williams, & Steveley, 1984; Sprague, & Horner, 1984) to severely handicapped persons. The previous investigations of general case instruction primarily utilized consecutive nontrained probes of an instructional universe following the attainment of training criteria on the selected teaching examples. Therefore, untrained probes were used as the sole dependent measure while training data were not presented graphically. Although performance on probe measures of an instructional universe may be the preferred dependent variable in general case instruction (Horner, 1982), the procedure fails to indicate a concurrent relationship between training and probe measures. Alternatively, nontrained probe measures may be provided during training to verify the ongoing effects of training on generalized responses and to serve as an additional indicator of the attainment of training criteria (Giangreco, 1983; Woolcock, Lyon, & Woolcock, in press).

Using a procedure similar to general case instruction, Lloyd, Saltzman, and Kauffman (1981) combined preskills instruction on representative mathematical facts with a counting "attack strategy" (p. 204) to teach generalized multiplication and division skills to students with learning disabilities. The selection of teaching examples that sampled the range of possible one-digit multiplication and division problems allowed the students to learn the mathematical skills necessary to perform across the "continuous field" (Skinner, 1953) of stimulus variations present in the instructional universes for both skills. The procedure permitted a direct analysis of the students' generalized performance on permanent product measures and allowed measurement across a continuous field of stimuli. This type of measurement contrasts with general case applications in which the stimuli are presented in discrete, noncontinuous units, such as different types of vending machines (Sprague, & Horner, 1984).

To date, general case instruction has not been applied to persons with sensory handicaps, particularly visual impairments, nor has such instruction included the use of specialized adaptive devices for performing tasks. In the study described here, general case instruction was used to teach three visually impaired and moderately retarded adults to sort nine representative two-digit zip code prefixes (the first two zip code numbers). At the same time, probes were made of the subjects' performance without training on the continuous field of zip code prefixes in the instructional universe of 100 U.S. zip code prefixes similar to those encountered when sorting national nonprofit mailing contracts. The ability to maintain and extend these sorting skills on the probes and mailing contracts was measured for two subjects during the final phases of the study.

Method

Subjects and setting

Three adults who were enrolled in a work-activities center for persons with visual impairments and multiple handicaps participated in the study. Vernon was a 53-year-old man with less than 20/200 vision, a severe-to-profound sensory neural hearing loss, and moderate mental retardation. Because of Vernon's deafness, the instructors used American sign language instead of verbal prompts during the study. Gail was a 44-year-old woman with Down syndrome who had less than 20/200 vision and moderate mental retardation. Mike was a 28-year-old man with Down syndrome, less than 20/200 vision and moderate mental retardation. All three subjects required a 10x magnifier in addition to corrective lenses to read typewritten print.

Before the study, each subject had attained proficiency in sorting mail by the last two digits corresponding to the final zip code numbers in a large metropolitan area (20 variations). Therefore, the aim of the study was to teach them to expand this ability in sorting national zip codes by their first two digits.

All instructional and nontrained probe sessions were conducted in the vocational production area at the work-activities center. Materials were arranged on two large work tables in a separate section of the production area.

Materials
Instructional and nontrained probe materials consisted of the following items:
1. A 66 inch (167.64cm) by 44 inch (111.76cm) sheet of plywood on which 121, 4 inch (10.16cm) by 6 inch (15.64cm) sorting rectangles were marked, placed across two work tables as a sorting board.
2. Twenty, 3 inch (7.62cm) by 5 inch (12.70cm) note cards were glued to the top and left sides of the sorting board and

were used as cue cards. Ten first-digit cue cards, divided into five sections, were marked with the first digits (0-9, 1 inch [2.54cm] high) in the first section of each card and were placed serially across the tops of each vertical column. Similarly, 10 second-digit cue cards were marked with second digits in the second section and were placed serially down the left side of each horizontal column (see Figure 1).
3. General case instructional sets of 45, 3 inch (7.62cm) by 5 inch (12.70cm) note cards with full addresses and zip codes (typed in IBM Delegate) were provided for each subject. The first two digits of each card corresponded to three inital-, three medial-, and three final-order zip codes for each subject. The subjects received instruction using 5 cards for each of the following assigned prefixes: Vernon, 11, 14, 17, 41, 44, 47, 71, 74, 77; Gail, 22, 25, 28, 52, 55, 58, 82, 85, 88; and Mike, 33, 36, 39, 63, 66, 69, 93, 96, 99.
4. A nontrained probe set of 500, 3 inch (7.62cm) by 5 inch (12.70cm) note cards with full mailing addresses (typed in IBM Delegate) was used for all subjects. Five different cards were used for each of the 100 zip code spaces.

Procedures

General case instruction
The three subjects received individual instruction on five fully addressed cards

for each of their nine assigned representative zip code prefixes. During the instructional sessions, the instructor first demonstrated the sorting of one card for each of the nine general case prefixes by 1) matching the first zip code digit to the corresponding digit at the top of the proper vertical column, 2) matching the second digit to the corresponding digit on the cue card at the left side of the proper horizontal column, or 3) placing the card in the correct section of the sorting board. A shuffled set of 45 individualized instructional cards was then given to the subject, accompanied by the verbal prompt (signed prompt for Vernon), "Sort these cards by the first two zip code numbers."

When a subject placed a card incorrectly, the instructor used a "least intrusive prompts strategy" (Snell, 1983) in providing a hierarchy of correctional procedures that included 1) a verbal prompt (signed to Vernon), "Try another space," 2) a gesture (pointing to the correct space), and 3) physical guidance (a hand-over-hand prompt to place the card in the correct space). Correct placement and incorrect placement (that required assistance) were recorded on a frequency/event data sheet with five spaces for recording a plus or minus to correspond to each zip code prefix.

Nontrained probes
During baseline and weekly probe sessions, each subject was presented with a

	0	1	2	3	4	5	6	7	8	9
0										
1		Vernon			Vernon			Vernon		
2			Gail			Gail			Gail	
3				Mike			Mike			Mike
4		Vernon			Vernon			Vernon		
5			Gail			Gail			Gail	
6				Mike			Mike			Mike
7		Vernon			Vernon			Vernon		
8			Gail			Gail			Gail	
9				Mike			Mike			Mike

Figure 1. Diagram of the sorting board. The first digits on the cue cards are at the top, and the second digits on the cue card are on the left side. Instructional prefixes are delineated by the subjects' names, which were not included on the actual sorting box.

shuffled probe set of 500 fully addressed cards, 5 for each prefix. The instructor initiated the probe sessions with the prompt, "Sort these cards by the first two numbers" (signed to Vernon), following which the subjects sorted cards into their corresponding spaces, without the instructor's intervention, during the 1-hour and 2 ¼ -hour probe periods allotted for each probe measure. Frequency/event data were recorded by indicating a plus for the correct placement or a minus for the incorrect placement of each card during the time that was allotted or for the complete sorting of the 500-card probe set.

Experimental design

During all the nontrained probe and instructional phases, a single-subject, multiple baseline experimental design across subjects (Baer, Wolf, & Risley, 1968) was used that incorporated a multiple probe technique (Horner, & Baer, 1978) (see figure 2). This design allowed for experimental control through measurement of the effects of the sequential introduction of general case instruction, contrasted with extended baseline probe measures across the three subjects. Data collected during each instructional and probe session were converted to the percentage of accurate sorts by the two-digit zip code prefix by dividing the number of correct placements by the total number of placements and multiplying by 100. Experimental sessions were sequenced according to the following experimental phases:

Baseline probe

Each subject was individually assigned to sort the 500-card probe set during one-hour baseline probe sessions. Frequency/event data were recorded according to each subject's initial nontrained correct and incorrect performance on 45 cards included in each subject's designated nine representative zip code prefixes (in the 500-card probe set) and the entire 500-card probe set.

General case instruction/one-hour probe

Individual instructional sessions incorporated a least-intrusive prompts strategy combined with the collection of frequency/event data on 5 cards for each of the designated 9 zip code prefixes. In addi-tion, one-hour weekly probe sessions were conducted on the 500-card probe set to measure the subjects' generalized performance on 100 variations in the zip code prefixes.

Second probe phase

Following the general case instruction 1-hour probe phase, 2 ¼ -hour probes were conducted to determine the subjects' performance on the 500-card probe set without the time constraints imposed during the 1-hour probe sessions in the previous phase. Procedures for Vernon were varied in this phase because of his poor generalized performance during the previous 1-hour probes.

Maintenance probe

Maintenance probes were conducted at bi-weekly intervals following the completion of the 2 ¼ -hour probe phase to determine whether Gail and Mike had maintained their generalized sorting skills after an extended period without training or practice in sorting the national zip codes. Again, the procedures used with Vernon were varied in an attempt to improve his generalized performance.

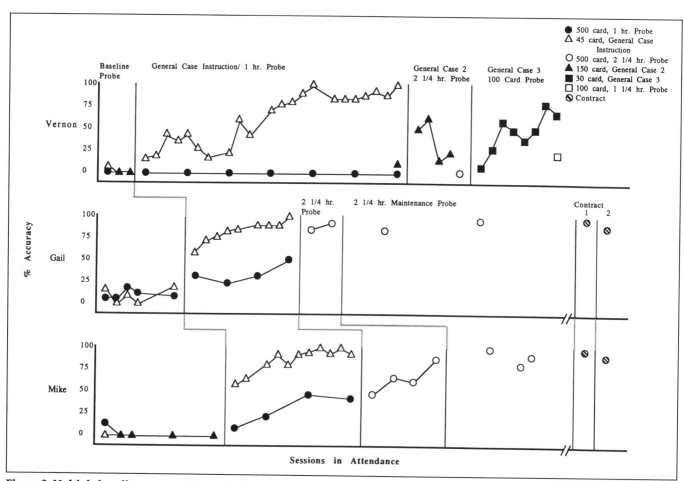

Figure 2. Multiple baseline across subjects design. Percentage of accuracy in sorting by the first two digits (prefix) of zip codes.

Contracts

The performance of Gail and Mike in sorting the 2 inch (5.05cm) by 3 inch (7.62cm) mailing labels in two national mailing contracts were assessed two months after the 2¼-hour maintenance probe phase. Gail and Mike each sorted the labels used in a 217-label contract and a 66-label contract.

Results

Interobserver reliability

Two observers independently scored separate data sheets according to the plus-or-minus scores for all the cards sorted by all three subjects during at least two sessions on the instructional and probe measures in each phase. Interobserver agreements were scored when both data sheets indicated the same number of correctly and incorrectly placed cards for each particular prefix; for example, when both data sheets indicated three correct and two incorrect cards in a prefix, five agreements were recorded. Disagreements were scored according to the disparity between the observers' scores for a particular prefix by counting the number of differing plus-or-minus scores. The percentage of interobserver agreement was derived by dividing the number of agreements by the number of agreements plus disagreements and multiplying by 100. The percentage of agreement on all measures ranged from 87 percent to 100 percent, with a mean of 96 percent for all instructional sessions and a mean of a 99 percent for all probe sessions.

Acquisition and generalized sorting

In the baseline probe phase, Vernon randomly placed 5 of the 45 general case instruction probe cards correctly during the first baseline probe session and failed to place any cards correctly in the two remaining sessions. His subsequent performance on the 45 designated general case instruction cards during general case instruction improved slowly, and he eventually attained complete accuracy. Despite his improved performance during general case instruction, he did not improve in the weekly one-hour probes of the 500-card probe set. Indeed, his performance during seven probe sessions did not improve at all, and he evidenced a great deal of frustration over the overwhelming number of cards to be sorted and the slow speed at which he performed the task. These factors appeared to affect Vernon's motivation to perform. Therefore, even with preferred reinforcers (coffee, cigarette breaks, and the like), Vernon's desire to perform the task accurately did not increase during the weekly probes.

Because of the deficits in Vernon's generalized performance, a second general case instruction phase was instituted in which 5 cards for each zip code beginning with 1, 4, and 7 (150 cards) were selected as instructional examples. The baseline probe of Vernon's performance on this 150-card set on the last day of the general case instruction/1-hour probe phase indicated that he correctly sorted 5 percent of the 150-card set in a nontrained probe. His performance on the 150-card set during instruction reached a high of 50 percent in the second instructional session but decreased during the final two instructional sessions. A 2¼-hour probe that was administered after the fourth instructional session indicated that Vernon did not generalize sorting skills after instruction on the 150-card set. Therefore, an alternative strategy was devised in which Vernon received instruction on a 30-card set and a prefix set of 1 card for each 1, 4, and 7 prefix, combined with weekly probes of a 100-card set with 1 card for each of the 100 zip code prefixes. The result of this strategy was a steady improvement in the acquisition of skills, but Vernon's generalized performance on concurrent probes was only 20 percent accurate.

Gail and Mike each performed with less than 25 percent accuracy in all baseline probe sessions. These baseline performances contrasted with their steady improvement during the general case instruction/one-hour probe phase in which both Gail and Mike's performance accelerated rapidly in successive general case instruction sessions and steadily but not as rapidly in concurrent weekly one-hour probe sessions.

The measurement of Gail's and Mike's accuracy during the final two 1-hour probe sessions revealed that all the cards that Gail and Mike had placed were accurate and that their levels of accuracy were low because they did not place most of the 500 cards on the board. Therefore, a 2¼-hour probe phase was instituted to provide the subjects with sufficient time to sort all 500 cards. In this phase, Gail's accuracy was 87 percent and 100 percent on consecutive probes, and she completed all cards before the end of the sessions. Although, Mike had difficulty remaining awake during the first three probes, he completed all cards and performed accurately on 80 percent of the cards in the final probe. Two weeks after her final 2¼-hour probe, Gail was administered a 2¼-hour maintenance probe (Mike was on vacation), and an additional probe was administered two weeks later; she performed with 87 percent and 94 percent accuracy on these two maintenance probes. When Mike returned from vacation, he was administered three 2¼-hour maintenance probes on which he performed accurately 96 percent, 74 percent, and 90 percent of the time. Two months after the 2¼-hour maintenance probe phase was completed, the work-activities center received two contracts to package and mail national mailings. Gail and Mike were each assigned to work the 2 inch (5.08cm) by 3 inch (7.62cm) labels for the 217-label and 66-label contracts using the sorting board. On these two mailings, their accuracy ranged from 83 percent to 96 percent.

Discussion

Results of the study described here document the effectiveness of general case instruction in producing a lasting increase in Gail's and Mike's generalized skills in sorting national zip codes. However, since Vernon did not demonstrate stable improved performance in his early general case instruction sessions or generalized sorting skills on probes, it may be questioned whether there was sufficient experimental control to compare Vernon's performance with Gail's and Mike's performances. Despite this discrepancy, the stable, rapidly improved performances of Gail and Mike indicated that sufficient experimental control existed within their baseline and treatment replications (Kazdin, 1978). Furthermore, the multiple treatment interference (Kratochwill, 1978) that was apparent across experimental phases was, in this instance, a desired cumulative effect of prior general case instruction and practice on probes. It resulted in Gail and Mike maintaining their skills even though it did not distinguish the effects of individualized treatments (instruction and probe practice) on generalized performance.

Procedural limitations

The 500-card probe set was selected because of the likelihood that the subjects would encounter such a large number of addresses in future mailing contracts. This number of cards limited the subjects' ability to complete the sorting of the cards in the allotted time and resulted in inadequate measures of generalization during the general case instruction/one-hour probe phase. The large probe set also decreased Vernon's (and, to some extent, Mike's) motivation to perform during probe sessions.

In light of these limitations, it is recommended that future replications of these or similar procedures should limit the number of examples in initial probe sets, possibly by beginning with 100 cards and increasing the number as students acquire speed and accuracy in the task. In reducing the number of probe cards, instructors may provide students with a greater opportunity to experience initial success and may reduce the potential for failure in the future that is inherent in the introduction of a large number or probe examples at the beginning of probe sessions.

The use of 500 probe cards also limited the ability of the data collectors to determine the common errors of the subjects because data collection was such a burdensome task that analyses were not feasible. This factor affected the investigators' ability to determine whether errors commonly occurred on zip code variations that were adjacent to those included in the general case instruction or whether they occurred on variations that were never included in the general case instruction (for example, all variations beginning with 0). It is possible that such an analysis with a 100-card probe set would determine whether more common errors occurred on "near-transfer" or "far-transfer items" (Lloyd, Saltzman, & Kaufman, 1981, p. 209), and might be useful in determining whether correct responses cluster around instructional variations in the continuous field of 100 variations.

Implications

In spite of the aforementioned limitations, the study provided evidence that general case procedures may be an efficient, effective method of teaching visually impaired and multiply handicapped persons to perform sophisticated tasks that include a larger number of stimulus and response variations. Indeed, before the study, no attempt had been made to teach the sorting of all 100 variations. Thus, the performance of this task had been restricted to those persons who could perform the task without instruction.

The study also provided an initial indication that the use of concurrent probes to assess generalization may supply valuable information about the ongoing impact of general case instruction on the performance of desired overall tasks. Although the probe set in the study was too large to allow the subjects to complete the task, their increasing levels of accuracy during the one-hour probes permitted the investigators to base their decision to terminate the general case instruction on data that showed the subjects' improved performance during general case instruction and during the one-hour probes. Subsequent investigations may expand the use of probes as criterion measures of the subjects' ability to generalize, particularly when measuring the generalized performance of community behaviors that result from stimulated general case instruction (see, for example, Woolcock, Lyon, and Woolcock, in press).

The results of the study expand the body of knowledge on the use of general case instruction in community, school, and vocational settings. The use of these procedures with visually impaired and multiply handicapped persons may be extended to include instruction in the areas of mobility skills (Horner, Jones, & Williams, 1985), community living skills (McDonnell, Horner, & Williams, 1984), and vocational skills (Horner & McDonald, 1982; Woolcock, Lyon, & Woolcock, in press). Through the use of general case procedures, instructors may use a minimum number of teaching examples to bring about enduring changes in functional behavior across a wide array of situations in which a particular behavior is expected to be performed.

References

Baer, D.M., Wolf, M.M. & Risley, T.R. (1968). Some current dimensions of applied behavior analysis. *Journal of Applied Behavior Analysis*, 1, 91-97.

Becker, W.C., & Engelmann, S. (1978). Systems for basic instruction: Theory and practice. In A.C. Catania and T.A. Brigham (Eds.), *Handbook of applied behavior analysis: Social and instructional processes* (pp. 325-377). New York: Irvington.

Giangreco, M.F. (1983). Teaching basic photography skills to a severely handicapped young adult using simulated materials. *Journal of the Association for the Severely Handicapped*, 8, 43-49.

Horner, R.D., & Baer, D.M. (1978). Multiple probe technique: A variation of the multiple baseline. *Journal of Applied Behavior Analysis*, 11, 189-196.

Horner, R.H. (1982, November). Teaching generalized behavior: Current research. Paper presented at the Ninth Annual Conference of the Association for the Severely Handicapped, Denver.

Horner, R.H., Jones, D.N., & Williams, J.A. (1985). A functional approach to teaching generalized street crossing. *Journal of the Association for Persons with Severe Handicaps*, 10, 71-78.

Horner, R.H., & McDonald, R.S. (1982). Comparison of single instance and general case instruction in teaching a generalized vocational skill. *Journal of the Association for the Severely Handicapped*, 7, 7-20.

Horner, R.H., Sprague, J., & Wilcox, B. (1982). General case programming for community activities. In B. Wilcox and G.T. Bellamy (Eds.), *Design of high school programs for severely handicapped students* (pp. 61-98). Baltimore: Paul H. Brookes.

Horner, R.H., Williams, J.A., & Steveley, J.D. (1984). Acquisition of generalized telephone use by students with severe mental retardation. Unpublished manuscript, University of Oregon, Eugene.

Kazdin, A.E., (1978). Methodology of applied behavior analysis. In A.C. Catania and T.A. Brigham (Eds.), *Handbook of applied behavior analysis: Social and instructional processes* (pp. 61-104). New York: Irvington.

Kratochwill, T.R. (1978). *Single subject research: Strategies for evaluating change.* New York: Academic Press.

Lloyd, J., Saltzman, N.J., & Kauffman, J.M. (1981). Predictable generalization in academic learning as a result of preskills and strategy training. *Learning Disability Quarterly*, 4, 203-216.

McDonnell, J.J., Horner, R.H., & Williams, J.A. (1984). Comparison of three strategies for teaching generalized grocery purchasing to high school students with severe handicaps. *Journal of the Association for Persons with Severe Handicaps*, 9, 123-133.

Skinner, B.F. (1953). *Science and human behavior.* New York: Macmillan Co.

Snell, M.E. (1983). Implementing the IEP: Intervention strategies. In M.E. Snell (Ed.), *Systematic instruction of the moderately and severely handicapped* (2nd ed., pp. 113-145). Columbus, OH: Charles E. Merrill.

Sprague, J.R., & Horner, R.H. (1984). The effects of single instance, multiple instance, and general case training on generalized vending machine machine use by moderately and severely handicapped students. *Journal of Applied Behavior Analysis*, 17, 273-278.

Woolcock, W.W., Lyon, S.R., & Woolcock, K.P. (in press). General case simulation instruction and the establishment and maintenance of work performance. *Research in Developmental Disabilities.*

William W. Woolcock, Ph.D., assistant professor, Teaching the Severely/Profoundly Handicapped Program, Department of Teacher Education, University of Arkansas, 33rd and University Avenue, Little Rock, AR 72204. Maureen Brody Lengel, M.Ed., Competitive Employment Opportunities, Pittsburgh, PA.

FUTURES

Although awareness of the needs and capabilities of those with multiple handicaps is increasing in the community at large, translation of that awareness into practice is still a primary challenge for the future. The closing article emphasizes four areas which require attention in order for the individual with multiple disabilities to achieve a satisfactory quality of life. With emphasis on advocacy, technological development, life planning, and professional preparation, individuals with multiple disabilities can participate more fully as members of the community.

Designing the Future: A Matter of Choice

J.N. Erin

For a child in contemporary society, the greatest challenge may be making effective choices. Life is no longer a predetermined route which moves from school to marriage to job and family. The myriad of options available to every child has only recently begun to evolve for children with special needs and for their families. For the multiply handicapped child, these options must continue to expand in education, living, and recreational settings in order to ensure the highest quality of life.

Recent data indicate increasing numbers of children with visual impairments and multiple disabilities (Gates, 1985). Medical innovations which sustain and prolong life, effects of chemical substances on newborns, and the continuing ebb and flow of disease and epidemic will continue to influence the presence of multiple disabilities and visual impairments among children and adults. Although the greatest hope of all professionals is that no child would have to experience disabilities, we know that this will not be the case in the near future.

To insure that children with multiple disabilities reach adulthood in a world which will allow them a satisfying quality of life, future planning must emphasize the development of advocacy, technology, life programming, and changing professional roles. In an era of community-based programming, one focus of the future will be on greater public involvement through advocacy efforts. Innovations in technology hold great promise for those with multiple disabilities. Life programming will replace the concept of education as a preparatory process for these individuals. Finally, changes in professional roles will be required in order to effectively implement life programming.

Advocacy

Advocacy is an artificial process. In an effective community, advocacy becomes unnecessary as an identified task: each community member advocates for himself and for others because each contributes to the total purpose of the community. Therefore, the end goal for advocacy with respect to low prevalence conditions is to make specific advocacy efforts by professionals unnecessary. In accomplishing this, advocacy should primarily become the role of the disabled individual and his family, but must also be regarded as the responsibility of the neighborhood and community. Given suitable resources and information, a community can provide an effective advocacy network with only short-term needs for external support.

There are two factors which impel us to advocate for the needs of the visually impaired individual with multiple handicaps: many such individuals do not have the skills to communicate their needs and concerns to the larger community; and the uniqueness of their disabilities makes it difficult for members of the general community to determine what is most important. However, our greatest dilemma as advocates is the fact that any statement of need based on the effects of disabilities connotes segregation . . . the need for a separate attention, service, or adaptation. Therefore, as advocates, we must not speak too loudly or too softly.

In order to be truly effective, the future in advocacy for the multiply handicapped individual with a visual impairment must encompass several areas. The first is a community focus. The emphasis for the multiply handicapped individual should not be on the effects of the disability but rather on that individual's potential as a member of the community. For some, that community may be an environment with other disabled individuals which relates to the surrounding neighborhood. For others, it may be the family and community in which they were raised; advocacy may mean assisting transition to an adult role in this setting.

The future role of the advocate will also be to provide accurate information, helping to separate fact from false belief. It is vital that information be publicly available to counteract common misunderstandings: "But why can't you just get an eye transplant?"; "But I heard about a boy like him who was blind and couldn't speak, and he turned out to be a musical genius!" Innovative medical and technological changes will continue to generate beliefs which are based on the hope that the disabled individual could be free of the disability. Advocacy must continue to focus on the value of the individual and not on the limitations implied by the physical condition.

A third vital function of advocacy will be communication with the medical community. Visually impaired individuals with multiple disabilities have sometimes been passed over as candidates for services which would enable them to use their vision most effectively. This can result from the difficulty of assessing an individual without a language system or from the common perspective that a severely handicapped person cannot use or benefit from corrective lenses and devices. Advocacy in this arena must take the form of a commitment to work with the medical system to achieve appropriate evaluation and correction. Accurate explanations and demonstrations of the individual's functional needs and learning processes will result in greater willingness of doctors to work toward optimal visual function.

Legislative advocacy will continue to be a priority among all groups and individuals concerned with disability. The recognition of the right of individuals with multiple disabilities to the opportunities afforded to all citizens will continue to be an objective. Assisting in the development of legislation which will accomplish this in the most cost-effective manner will be a primary goal in advocacy.

However, the most effective tool for advocacy in the future will be planning for successful outcomes. Examples of individuals with multiple disabilities who are living comfortable, balanced lifestyles are the most effective statements which can be made about other individuals with similar needs. Placement in a setting which is too restricted or too unstructured can generate frustration and can focus outside attention on an individual's limitations. A well-planned continuum which provides the multiply handicapped individual with needed skills and the opportunity to practice them will enable that person to be an advocate for others.

Technology

Within the last decade, technological innovations for disabled individuals have emerged and changed with kaleidoscopic speed. For the visually impaired individual, access to information has increased through rapid braille, large type, and speech output. Devices and software with single and multiple functions have become widely available, and the emphasis has shifted to the production of efficient materials at a reasonable cost.

Applications for the individual with physical disabilities and cognitive differences, however, require greater individualization. The recognition that technology can be valuable for those who may never be independent in the job market has come more slowly. Technological innovations may be the key to personal control in residential and community environments for many people with multiple handicaps and visual impairments; however, for this potential to be realized, attention must be given to several factors.

One such factor is the learning process related to the use of a technological device. Many devices hold promise for the individual with multiple disabilities, but the instructions and manuals are complex and are presented at a fixed level with respect to vocabulary, level of abstraction, and general structure. Attention to alternative learning processes which modify the quantity of information as well as maximize feedback to the user will facilitate access for those with various learning abilities.

Physical modifications are also necessary in making the best use of available technology. Many individuals with multiple handicaps and visual disabilities require adapted input and output options as well as creative applications of technology for work and life settings. Development of individualized modifications will require adequate funding which can be used flexibly and is not tied to a specific disability label. In addition, professional specialists who know the nature of disability as well as the capabilities of technology must be widely available and involved in program planning.

The expense and time involved in acquiring and using technology necessitates that long-term planning take place with the assurance of extensive application. It is inexcusable for a family to be encouraged to purchase a device which later proves too cumbersome, difficult, or inefficient for a child. It is equally frustrating for a device to be purchased which quickly becomes obsolete and is replaced by a more efficient model.

From the early years, a child's educational program should include skills which will enable him or her to take advantage of technological adaptations; however, the use of a device should be viewed as a means to an end rather than an end in itself. In our eagerness to overcome physical barriers, we must not rely on the use of a device as a destination but rather as a vehicle for achieving a goal. A child who can use a single device for assistance in a number of daily tasks has a greater advantage than one who can use a complex device for only one purpose.

The future in technology is promising for the multiply handicapped individual with visual impairments. Options such as speech output; self-programmed communication boards in which the user can devise the visual stimulus; and computer programs which rely on picture or rebus symbols rather than printed words are alternatives which may be useful to some visually impaired individuals. With careful planning and thorough evaluation, technology will continue to expand beyond the classroom and work setting.

Life programming

Our educational system is based on the notion that formal learning ought to take place early in life as a means of preparation for a career. Formal learning which takes place after that time is for the purpose of enrichment or career advancement. Only recently have we come to think of education as a process which can be lifelong.

For an individual with a visual disability and additional handicaps, this concept is an essential one. The presence of a visual disability alone limits the amount of information available to an individual; learning through tactual and auditory modes requires sequential processes, and time is the greatest deterrent to efficiency through these channels. If an individual also has a cognitive difference, slower learning rates and retention of less information will result. In combination, these two conditions imply the necessity for extended learning time. Although all individuals might profit from education beyond the growing years, this is a critical feature for those with multiple disabilities, from whom the environment requires greater adaptation.

The current emphasis on functional curriculum for the severely handicapped individual has implications for future life-skill planning. The importance of skill generalization across settings, people, and materials underscores the ultimate pragmatic function of education: it should focus on maximum independence in residential, vocational, and recreational settings and should continue well into adulthood for those who require it.

For the individual with multiple disabilities and a visual impairment, two factors are critical. One is the cooperative and efficient participation of support agencies in the planning process. In the past, we have relied on agencies which compartmentalized services according to the age of the individual involved. Future planning must provide for a flow of services within agencies so that transition takes place throughout life and is not patchwork intended to join two discrete stages. Early identification of a primary serving agency and specification of the roles of support agencies will make the planning process less cumbersome and territorial.

The other factor is the recognition of the family and the disabled individual as primary decision makers. In recent years, professionals have broadened their viewpoint from a family-training philosophy to one in which the family is viewed as a unit requiring broad-based support in order to provide optimally for the member with disabilities (Goetz, Guess, & Stremel-Campbell, 1987). This concept must be applied in future planning efforts; families must be encouraged to discuss their hopes and goals for the future and to realize these through early planning in order to provide adequately for all family members.

Professional preparation

The past decades have prepared professionals who have often seen their role as specialized. The greater the number of labels associated with a student or client, the more specialists were required. The emergence of the multidisciplinary team fostered the concept that the complexity of multiple disabilities required expertise beyond what one or two professionals could provide.

Although this approach has generally improved service delivery for multiply handicapped children, it has created risks in several areas which require future attention. A team which functions as a composite of specialists may leave students vulnerable to fragmented programming and territorial perspectives. As professionals, we have often reenacted "The Blind Man and the Elephant," perceiving only one area of need or function rather than setting priorities which are appropriate for the total individual.

Economic necessity may be the rod that goads us to restructure professional roles. The inefficiency of operating as a collection of experts has become apparent, particularly with respect to children with multiple handicaps and visual impairments. In order for a child to learn effectively, there must be an individual who is clearly responsible for program implementation and who has received intensive preparation to do so. While the team will continue to be vital for effective programming, the role of the team leader and the methods for effective implementation of goals must receive greater emphasis.

This poses a special challenge to the colleges responsible for teacher preparation. They must produce intensively prepared educators to serve a group which comprises a minute fraction of the school-aged population. This will require intensive programs at a few key sites nationally which can combine teacher preparation with research in practice. It will require flexible options such as summer workshops and outreach courses which will meet personnel needs in rural areas.

In addition, future preparation must regard alternative roles, particularly those in direct care. The paraprofessional is fre-quently the individual who spends the most time in contact with a visually impaired individual with multiple handicaps, and yet few programs which prepare paraprofessionals include even basic information on severe disabilities and visual impairments. It is vital that community college programs be expanded to present information specific to this population. In addition, the paraprofessional role must be recognized as a vital one in effective programming; teaching practice and course-work must include experience in working with paraprofessionals.

Finally, preparing effective professionals will require support for research specific to the needs of the person with multiple handicaps and visual disabilities. While our current approaches combine best practices in work with severely handicapped people and visually impaired individuals, we have little to guide us with respect to those with both disabilities. Particularly with respect to vision usage, we still lack broad-based information about the learning processes of children with specific conditions such as cortical visual impairment. Federal support for research in this area will continue to be critical to the development of knowledge about best instructional practice.

The key to an optimal quality of life for the person with multiple disabilities and a visual impairment lies in the four areas of advocacy, technology, life programming, and professional preparation. With advancement in each of these areas, the future will provide an array of choices for these individuals and will create greater opportunities for each individual to make those choices. Only in this way can families and communities support the role of the individual with multiple disabilities as a contributing member of the system.

References

Gates, C. (1985). Survey of multiply handi-capped visually impaired children in the Rocky Mountains/Great Plains region. *Journal of Visual Impairment & Blindness, 79*, 385-391.

Goetz, L., Guess, D., & Stremel-Campbell, K. (1987). *Innovative program design for individuals with dual sensory impairments.* Baltimore: Paul H. Brookes.

Jane N. Erin, Ph.D., assistant professor, Programs for the Education of the Visually Handicapped, The University of Texas at Austin, Education Bldg. 306, Austin, TX 78712-1290.